How to Live With

PTSD

The Causes and Characteristics of

POST TRAUMATIC STRESS DISORDER

Beverly J. Peterson, Ph.D., MSN, RN, MFT
Richard W. Peterson, Ph.D., MBA

ISBN 0-9634079-3

How to Live with PTSD
Causes and Characteristics

Copyright 2000 by
Beverly Peterson, RN, MS, MFT, Ph.D and
Richard Peterson MBA, Ph.D
Second printing May 2003

Published by
    Consultors Incorporated
    1285 Rubenstein Avenue
    Cardiff by the Sea, California 92007

Printed in the United States of America.
All rights reserved under International and Pan American Copyright Conventions.
No part of this book may be reproduced or transmitted in any form or by any means, electronic or mechanical, including photocopying, recording, or by any information storage and retrieval system, without written permission of the authors.
ISBN 0-9634079-3-7

How to Live With
PTSD

TABLE OF CONTENTS	PAGE
PREFACE	i
CHAPTER ONE - POST TRAUMATIC STRESS DISORDER	1
CHAPTER TWO – CHARACTERISTICS	29
CHAPTER THREE – CAUSES	75
CHAPTER FOUR –COPING	97
CHAPTER FIVE - CASES	127
APPENDIX 1	159
REFERENCES	163
SUBJECT INDEX	165

INTRODUCTION

We wrote this book to answer the many questions we get from clients and other therapists regarding the manifold symptoms and effect of Post Traumatic Stress Disorder. It is not intended to substitute for professional help in the case of those who suffer with Post Traumatic Stress Disorder. The insight and help that psychotherapists offer is vitally needed by anyone who lives with the tragic aftermath of trauma. We urge anyone with the symptoms of PTSD to consult their therapist.

Dr. Beverly Peterson is a counseling therapist with more than twenty five years experience in psychotherapy. Her career began as a Lieutenant in the US Navy where, during the Viet Nam War era, she served as a psychiatric nurse. She continues her private practice of psychotherapy as a licensed Marriage Family Therapist.

Dr. Richard Peterson is a counseling therapist. He spent a number of years as a Readjustment Counselor with the Department of Veterans Affairs in the Vet Center system. of the Veterans Administration. During WWII as an infantry sergeant in Germany, his entire regiment was surrendered by its commander, and he became a prisoner of war.

This book is the result of our personal experience, empirical evidence and academic research. It is our sincere hope that therapists and the casualties from PTSD they serve will find it helpful.

Beverly J. Peterson, RN, MS, MFT, Ph.D.
Richard W. Peterson, Ph.D., MBA

PREFACE

Our inability to recognize PTSD is surprising in view of the many traumatic incidents observed by the medical profession over the years. We know that war created mental damage and that it was ignored once the battles ended. No one ever appeared to connect the post trauma problems from warfare with the post trauma problems in civilians. The "Nostalgia" of the American Civil War soldier and the "Railroad disease" of mid 19th century Britain, later determined to be PTSD apparently were ignored in dealing with the trauma of World War I and certainly World War II and Korea.

During the First World War, Captain W. H. Rivers was a medical officer at the Craiglockhart War Hospital in England. These extracts are from an address he made to the Royal Society of Medicine on Dec. 4th, 1917, and published in the Lancet February 2, 1918. The title of his address was "The Repression of War Experience." Rivers was on the right track in treating the problem, but he did not understand the complexity of the experience, or the long-term effects of what we now call PTSD.

His definition of the term repression was "the active or voluntary process by which it is attempted to remove some part of the mental content out of the field of attention with the aim of making it inaccessible to memory and producing the state of suppression." Doctors at the time seemed to think that a person could consciously force a state of amnesia. Patients were advised to put all thoughts of war from their minds. He maintained the problems faced by the returning soldier were the result of failed repression. The memories continued to return if the repression was unsuccessful.

He went on to say, "It's not the repression itself which is harmful, but repression under conditions in which it fails to adapt the individual to his environment." While it was felt that a person could actively repress memories, the inability to adapt created the painful and intrusive memories that caused the mental disturbance. Now we realize that the unconscious mind holds these memories. By doing that, it causes a reaction to outside stimuli based on these memories.

Rivers disagreed in part with this prevailing theory. It was his opinion that if the sufferer could discuss the traumatic experience in a rational manner, it would become less frightening. The patient would no longer look at the experience from a twisted memory. This method was a precursor of our re-framing the trauma. We attempt now to get the sufferer to look at the traumatic event in as rational and realistic a manner as possible.

He quotes from a number of cases. One patient had successfully avoided thoughts of war while he was awake. In dreams they came back vividly, causing sleeplessness. When the patient discussed his experiences with Dr. Rivers, and uncovered the resultant anxieties, his sleeplessness disappeared.

Today this is the accepted form of therapy. We get the patient to remember the bad experiences as realistically as possible. This effort removes the mental fog in which repulsive memories are surrounded. When this is accomplished, the person no longer looks at events distorted by the trauma. This is not to suggest the memory is removed, or that the effect of the incident is eliminated. Rather the unrealistic fear is displaced.

One case presented by Dr. Rivers was of an officer who discovered the mangled body of his best friend. In his dreams the corpse would return, coming closer and closer, making the officer flee until he woke trembling and in a sweat. Rivers was successful in getting the officer to change the dream. In the revised dream, when he discovered his friend's body, he knelt by it to pray, and remove his personal effects for return to his family. He awoke from that new dream feeling grief and sadness for the loss of a friend. No trace of the horror remained.

Rivers termed this effort "re-education." That is what we now call re-framing. In that effort we approach the trauma from another angle in an effort to make the memory more authentic. We eliminate the distortion brought into the picture by life before and after the event. Those feelings can so warp the truth of what happened that the memory becomes consciously unbearable. Terms to describe the event like awful, dreadful, repulsive, and unbearable come into play where they really are not appropriate.

The approaches Dr. Rivers took with these patients were not always successful. He related the case of a man who had successfully repressed all thoughts of war. Using solitude and isolation, he effectively was able to put all thoughts of combat out of his mind. While Rivers did not realize it, we now realize that the unconscious always hangs on to the disturbing memories. A remark or event totally unrelated to the memory would bring the effects of the trauma to the surface, with all of the upset and confusion of the original. Rivers was unable to counteract the reaction of the person's unconscious, which held the memory of the trauma.

This can also be the trigger for what we now define as intrusive memory. One who lives with PTSD can actively put thoughts of the trauma out of their mind, but the unconscious brings it back when it is triggered. Such a trigger does not have to be directly connected to the original trauma. It can be brought back by an odor, ambient temperature, conditions of darkness or light, a sound, or any one of many other stimuli that open the door to the unconscious.

Rivers went on to discuss the value of sharing as a cathartic for eliminating the exaggerated memories, what he termed re-education, and an element of faith. In today's therapy modality we try to get the client to discuss the traumatic experience in order to look at it realistically, and without the *mea culpa* feeling that many hold. In today's therapy efforts, we do all we can to bring the client to the point where acceptance for their part is realistically accepted. We do not mean to minimize the impact of traumatic events, but it is vital they be put into proper perspective. Reality is the only way to view such events if they are to be dealt with. Most therapists accept the idea of the element of faith. It is as simple as believing that a solution can and will be found for the misery of PTSD. The joined faith of the client and the therapist combined with their mutual effort often shows the way to alleviate the difficulties of the disorder.

Rivers recommended moderation in the effort to bring back painful memories. He said, "It is just as armful to dwell persistently upon painful memories or anticipation's and brood upon feelings of regret and shame, as to (attempt to) banish them wholly from the mind. " This recalls a recommendation in some of the current twelve step literature, where those with addictions are told to "Look at the past, but don't stare at it."

Freud presented his theories regarding the wartime super-ego a few years after the end of World War I. He hypothecated that the superego, our voice of conscience, is replaced by a wartime superego which recognizes that killing and destruction are acceptable behaviors. By this mental shift, civilian soldiers are able to reconcile their earlier training regarding rights of others to a peaceful existence, replaced by feeling that killing and raw personal survival without regard for others is proper conduct. At the end of hostilities, many men found discarding the war time superego with their peacetime superego was a terrible battle. Some lost, and never did recover. Others repressed the memories of their actions in war, only to discover they remained in their subconscious until they showed up as Post Traumatic Stress. As a result of his theory, Freud recommended that all military organizations should be made up of mercenaries, professional fighters. He felt the impact on the civilian soldier was too harmful to continue using them in wartime. He had two sons in the German Army during World War I. We can only speculate that he saw and was deeply disturbed by the personality changes in them after their military service.

Today we realize the long term effect of trauma. The early practitioners felt that once the memories ere put to rest the problem was resolved.

We no longer think this way. Thanks to the research of the early 1980's, and the continuing work since then to understand Post Traumatic Stress Disorder, we have developed some techniques to alleviate the torment of PTSD.

POST TRAUMATIC STRESS DISORDER
Causes, Characteristics, and Coping

CHAPTER ONE

A mysterious ailment came home with men who returned from Viet Nam. Lost in the anti-war demonstrations, discounted by the medical and psychological communities, and almost derided by many in the health care arena, the well hidden terrible mental damage they carried with them was ignored. Not for a decade would this problem be identified as Post Traumatic Stress Disorder.

These men and women returned to a country tired of war, controlled by their elders who were products of WWII and the Korean conflict. Military hospitals that were able to handle and heal the most egregious wounds were unable to understand their complaints. Military superiors took the attitude that now that the guns were silent, any complaints that did not involve physical damage were charged up to malingering. The military establishment completely ignored the fact that an estimated 300,000 veterans of World War II suffered from some sort of mental disorder brought on by their service.

As the civilian soldiers were slowly discharged into the civilian community, their complaints fell on deaf ears. Labeled as cry babies, most learned to keep their problems to themselves. Career military people did the same for fear of damaging their positions and promotions.

In the civilian world many suffered with anxiety and nervous disorders brought on by natural disasters such as earthquake, flood, tornadoes, and fire. Other tragedies caused trauma. Automobile accidents, other sudden death events, shipwreck, drowning, murder, aircraft crashes, riots, and other dangers beyond any person's control caused trauma to those who had never seen a combat zone.

It seems reasonable to assume that because of the concentration of people in the military service and patients in the Veterans Hospitals the solution to this real problem was defined by those working in these areas. As the disorder became better understood, it became obvious that it affected more than those who had served in the military.

Men and women with Post Traumatic Stress Disorder have a lot of problems in their lives. They suffer with a multitude of issues with various common symptoms in varying combinations. Most have problems sleeping and nightmares when sleeping. Many live with flashbacks, the unexplained phenomenon when a person has a powerful feeling that he or she is reliving the time of their trauma. Try as they might, they continue to re-experience the fear and terror of the event. They feel more comfortable being alone, but are disturbed by the fact that they do not seem to get along well with people. The complaint is that people don't really understand them. One of the most debilitating symptoms is the feeling of "What's the use?" which slows or stops progress on their life path. Mistrust of institutions or organizations is almost endemic in this group of people who have lived through trauma. They are hyper alert. Often this hyper alertness moves on into full blown paranoia, where the subject feels everyone is out to get them. With hyper alertness comes an exaggerated startle response. Often they use the term "jumpy." Abuse of alcohol or drugs is a symptomatic outgrowth of PTSD, but is not part of the symptomatic description even though it is wide spread.

They do not want to think of the time, place or circumstances surrounding the trauma. They avoid talking and thinking about it, and avoid any thing or person that would remind them of the time of the trauma. Those who have lived through trauma have difficulty becoming close to another human. They have difficulty with emotions, especially those involving tenderness, love and sexuality. Multiple affairs, and or divorce and remarriage are common. Domestic quarrels, with spouses and children are prevalent fueled by drunkenness or drug abuse. Because of what is called psychic numbing, those with PTSD find little joy in normal activities or even in life itself.

The symptoms of the disorder are often held in check for an extended period of time. We find that it comes to the fore when there should be less stress in a person's life. They appear when children are grown and gone, when financial problems are resolved, and in times of a tranquil family life and good health. This is not to say there has not been evidence of some problem before this time, but the so called middle years are fertile ground for the disorder to take on a disturbing intensity.

There is hope to minimize the after affects of trauma. Modern psychology has helped many to find peace of mind even though the memories of their traumas remain. What is accomplished is an understanding and methods of turning the flame of trauma into manageable ashes of memory.

PTSD, Post Traumatic Stress Disorder results from experiencing or witnessing an event outside the range of usual human experience that would be markedly distressing to almost anyone, according to the Diagnostic and Statistical Manual of Mental Disorders. Except in its most debilitating form the sufferer often ignores PTSD. In that regard, it is like hypertension, showing few symptoms until the system overloads. This "lie in the weeds" characteristic has caused many misdiagnoses, and a lot of personal unhappiness.`

WHAT IS TRAUMA, AND HOW DOES IT HAPPEN?

Trauma is the reaction to exposure to an extreme stressor. It involves the personal experience of an event that could cause actual or threatened death, serious injury, or some other threat to one's physical integrity. It could result from witnessing an event that involves death, injury, or a threat to the physical integrity of another person, particularly one who is closely related by blood, marriage, or friendship. Trauma can result from learning about unexpected or violent death, serious harm, or threat of death or injury experienced by a family member or other close associate

The symptoms of PTSD are not obvious. Those who have endured a trauma serious enough to cause the disorder do not exhibit apparent symptoms to the casual observer. The family lives with personality traits difficult to understand. Spouses particularly are subjected to the mood swings, the unpleasant results of substance or alcohol abuse, the sleepless nights, or the recurring nightmares. They wonder about the lack of emotional closeness, the seeming dearth of ambition, or the constant changing of jobs. They wonder why long range plans for the family are an anathema and if made, are seldom followed to completion. That those with PTSD like to be alone; to avoid social contact is a common character trait. The family learns to leave the one with PTSD alone or suffer the anger resulting from the interruption. The fears brought on by paranoia, the keeping of firearms which they will say is the result of concern for family safety, or the suspicion toward institutions (particularly government), are so much a part of the sufferers personality, they become a tolerable, although unpleasant part of their lives. These personality characteristics develop slowly. They do not spring full-grown shortly after a trauma occurs. They develop slowly, an outgrowth of the event. Because they do not show up for months or years after the trauma happened, often the victim does not connect the trauma to present day problems.

Many who live with PTSD seem fully functional until they react to unknown stimuli. Then the long suppressed suffering comes to consciousness with all of the horror, pain and agony of the original trauma. The anxiety and depression returns. When those with PTSD consult psychiatrists, psychotherapists, counselors, or discuss their feelings with friends and family, their distress is often mistaken for anxiety, depression, paranoia, and even bi-polar disorders. Those who lived with PTSD in the military were often suspected of malingering.

Post Traumatic Stress Disorder (PTSD) is a frightening, frustrating and debilitating mental disorder. It lies just below the surface, causing disruptions in the life of the sufferer. Some of the results of PTSD include not wanting to be close to others, feelings of being an outsider, of sleeplessness, and addictions. To the family or co-worker, the strange and unpredictable actions and reactions of the one who lives with Post Traumatic Stress Disorder are upsetting and annoying.

These are some of the cases we have seen:

Sam Cass served as a Navy Corpsman with the Marines during the Viet Nam war. Twenty years later he continues to wake up screaming from the nightmare of seeing men destroyed by rockets and mortars. The terrible feelings of inability to save all of the wounded return with unimaginable intensity.

Dorothy Paul adores her husband, but cannot respond to his love making because of a date rape while a college freshman. While she cannot remember specifics of the rape, her aversion is an unwanted powerful restriction to a loving relationship.

Robert Frank awakens in a sweat from his dream of the din, dirt and flying glass that surrounded him in the automobile wreck that killed his two best friends. He was driving the car. He does not remember the immediate physical pain, masked by shock, but the horror returns, intensified by his feelings of guilt.

Ben Short watched in silent horror as the home he and his wife built exploded in the flames of a firestorm. The gut-wrenching sense of loss comes back in waves of memory when he least expects it.

Even though they live in different cities, are of varying ages, education, race and occupation, Sam Cass, Dorothy Paul, Robert Frank, and Ben Short all have one thing in common. They experience the agony of Post Traumatic Stress Disorder. PTSD respects no one regardless of age, income, social or educational level. It can hit anyone. One common denominator is the experiencing a sense of great, personal, unrecoverable loss.

PTSD is the strange and complicated mental disorder that confused practitioners for a number of years in spite of a centuries old history replete with victims who suffered from it by different names. The earliest diagnosis was called "Railroad Disease." During the early days of rail transport in Britain, accidents were much more common because of the relatively primitive equipment and trackage in use versus that of today. Months after being involved in a railway accident, many people found themselves nervous, irritable, frightened, and suffering from a general mental discomfort.

Men who abandoned their front line posts to return home during the War Between the States in the 1860's were said to be suffering from "nostalgia." No doubt many were convicted for desertion, but in those apparently more gentle days, the failings of men otherwise brave and gallant were excused more easily. Little is written about the long term effects of "nostalgia," but the description of it as an indeterminate mental malaise indicates it was a type of Post Traumatic Stress Disorder.

In the First World War when combat soldiers became mentally disturbed, their problem was diagnosed as "shell shock" because war had never before subjected men to the intense artillery barrages of both sides during 1914-1918. The simplistic idea was that the intense noise and dirt created by an artillery attack would destroy the mental stability of otherwise good soldiers. Except for Freud's concept the peacetime consequences of a wartime superego, no one pursued the long term affects on the doughboys of WWI.

World War II produced battle fatigue, made most famous by an unknown soldier being slapped by a popular general who believed men were either heroes or cowards. The general had no use for a soldier not being on the line as long as he was not bleeding. Studies made at the end of World War II, kept secret by the War Department until recent years, indicate about 30% (about 300,000) of combat soldiers were suffering from battle fatigue at the end of the war. In 1980, some 35 years after the end of the largest war in history, the first encompassing survey of former soldiers was done, but the data for the previous three decades was lost to the statisticians and psychologists.

Not until 1980, five years after the end of the vicious fighting in Viet Nam, was the term PTSD applied to the men who had brought home the many facets of Post Traumatic Stress Disorder. They had been misdiagnosed, maltreated, and often abandoned by the medical profession for at least a decade because no one could agree on a diagnosis, much less a treatment. Much treatment reflected the feelings of the WWII general so it was less than effective.

In 1980 this complex disorder was finally properly defined. New studies continue to discover its many sources. The existence of PTSD is often completely missed by mental health practitioners who do not often observe it. Many sufferers continue to live unhappily with subdued anger, frustration, and fear, unaware they carry in their subconscious the smoldering embers of their traumas. Those embers can erupt into a raging fire in a split second, causing uncontrolled reactions to the unconscious memories of the trauma.

PTSD: WHERE DOES IT COME FROM?

Post Traumatic stress disorder is the result of seeing or being involved in an event far outside our usual human experience. It involves being involved in a disastrous situation over which you had no control. Such horrifying and terrifying events either caused, or could have caused death or great injury to you or someone close to you. Your reaction was one of great fear and feelings of helplessness.

The effects of PTSD have been known for centuries. Recently the disorder has been more clearly defined. Previously, the wartime disorder was given other labels. Now we recognize that PTSD affects many that were never in a war zone. Witnessing or being involved in any kind of traumatic event can cause PTSD.

Experiences that can cause Post Traumatic Stress Disorder, include being in an automobile accident; living through an earthquake or a serious fire; surviving an airplane or train crash; living through a shipwreck; being caught up in a riot, or an out of control crowd situation. Being raped; being attacked by animals; finding yourself the target of an indiscriminate shooting, or being involved in an armed holdup; working as a paramedic; serving as a nurse or doctor in an emergency room; discovering a victim of suicide; and living through armed combat are all sources of PTSD. PTSD can result in those who have been mugged, physically assaulted, or who have discovered a close friend or relative has a terminal disease. One who has discovered a suicide or those who were concentration camp inmates, prisoners of war, or held hostage all live with the effects of PTSD. From combat the incidence of PTSD among front line medics was as high as that of the armed combatants.

Those in positions of responsibility for others are often victims. Police, paramedics, firefighters, rear echelon military commanders, sailors on a ship that foundered, airline personnel will live with a distorted sense of their responsibility to others that have seen suffer trauma. They too, will suffer with the effects of

PTSD. More so in these occupations, because they must continue to function even in the most adverse of conditions.

Traumatic events that cause a post trauma disorder are all beyond usual human experience. They often involve lightning-quick, and life threatening happenings. Those who are caught up in fire, earthquake, shipwreck, auto accidents, witnessing death and destruction, also often carry an attitude of innocence. Even the combat soldier feels a vulnerability and guilt based on childhood teaching of respect for life. Others doing their chosen jobs are impacted by traumas not of their making, whether they are the victim, an observer, or become a caregiver. The reaction is "Why is this happening to me?" With this feeling of disbelief the psyche mysteriously allows them to forget the intensity of the trauma soon after the event. We know this psychological defense mechanism offers relief from the tragedy. The trauma remains deeply implanted in the unconscious. Trauma has been likened to a subcutaneous cyst. While everything appears normal on the surface, beneath there is a hidden, serious infection.

Experiencing or observing a trauma creates a powerful impact on both our conscious and unconscious. The effects of the horror remain long after the happening. Even in the face of trauma, we apparently able to continue functioning. This is particularly obvious in the case of those involved in combat or areas of public safety. There is no time to mourn the loss of human life. We eliminate the event from our conscious memory in order to help and comfort the injured, and get on with the task at hand. We try to put the occurrence behind us so we can continue our lives. In our conscious mind we have done so, but the unconscious retains the pain and agony of the event. Post Traumatic Stress Disorder is a complex, confusing and disturbing mental ailment, primarily because it includes some elements of other mental disorders. Post Traumatic Stress Disorder is a recognized mental disorder, but it is also a collection of many other individual mental aberrations. PTSD shows evidence of paranoia, narcissism, addictive behavior, hysteria, many types of schizophrenia, particularly paranoia, selective amnesia, and egocentricity.

PTSD shatters our assumptions in these three areas:

1. Before trauma happens, there is a belief in personal invulnerability. We feel "it can't happen to me" so there is a lack of apprehension, of personal vulnerability, and a total disbelief that injury can happen.
2. We hold the perception that our private world is meaningful and comprehensible.
3. We lose earlier views of ourselves in a positive light. Then we held ourselves in high esteem, and felt we were worthy persons.

Think of Post Traumatic Stress Disorder in total, as a mobile sculpture. The whole sculpture moves when any part is touched. So if the person with Post Traumatic Stress Disorder has paranoiac thoughts, many of the other characteristics of the disorder are adversely stimulated. The clinical reactions to these other mental disturbances intensify the pain of PTSD in total. When paranoia or addictive behavior disturbs mental equilibrium, they spur the unpleasant and uncomfortable traumatic memories. The reactions are like hit and run mental torture. The pain is more intense than one would expect from the stimulus.

This is one case of a patient and his family, all of who lived with the confusion and disturbance that improperly diagnosis and treatment of PTSD can cause. Remember, the families of those who live with Post Traumatic Stress Disorder suffer a major part of the tragedy as well.

Arnold is an educated man holding an advanced degree from a fine university in the East. He is a sensitive, intellectual, caring individual, who was active in many activities with his family in school church and the community. In other words, a good family man. While serving in Viet Nam as a front-line infantryman, he was involved in heavy combat. The body count of the enemy was heavy. Many of his comrades suffered wounds or were killed. Among those killed, was Arnold's best friend. After Arnold's discharge from the Army, he sought medical and psychiatric help as the result of the traumas he suffered in Viet Nam. While the Viet Nam war ended in 1975, and in spite of historical evidence showing mental problems caused to those experiencing great trauma, the recognition of Post Traumatic Stress Disorder as a mental disorder did not evolve until 1980. Arnie was diagnosed as bi-polar, given medication for that disorder, and sent on his way. The doctors consistently adjusted his medication in futile efforts to give him some mental serenity.

After almost twenty years, his life became increasingly confusing. He found it became more and more difficult to work at his profession. The attendant financial difficulties created family problems. He came to us in an almost hysterical state. He was unable to work, his family life was disintegrating, he could not sleep, and his reaction to minor problems or incidents was that of an armed soldier. He was suspicious of others, and held strong feelings of being "different" than other men. He had persistent dreams of his best friend's death, and while there was no rationale for it, he was convinced he was totally responsible for the loss. Arnold and his family suffered with serious Post Traumatic Stress Disorder for two decades before anyone recognized the agony and disruption it was causing them individually and collectively.

DO I HAVE PTSD?

The diagnosis of PTSD or any other mental disorder is best left to the mental health professionals. However, it is our belief that the client knows the most about his or her feelings. If you are wondering if the difficulties in your life are the result of trauma, read through the following short descriptions to see if any of them fit your feelings and reactions to people, places and things. These characteristics describe some typical behavior as the result of Post Traumatic Stress Disorder.

1. If you have trouble sleeping at night because you can't stop the unformed fears—you may be suffering with Post Traumatic Stress Disorder.
2. If you wish everyone would go away and let you alone, but you are afraid of being alone—you may have PTSD.
3. If you avoid certain places because they make you uncomfortable, but you don't know why—you may be suffering with PTSD.

4. If certain situations remind you of a trauma in your life—it could be from the effects of PTSD.
5. If you feel as though you are wading through life in molasses, and can't get started with any interesting job or other activity---that could be PTSD.
6. If you cannot remember a traumatic time in your life that you thought you would never forget, PTSD has taken over your conscious memory.
7. If you wake up, and do not want to get out of bed because you can't think of a reason to do so—you may be living with the effects of a forgotten trauma—and that's PTSD.
8. If beginning something new--a project, a course of study, going on a trip, seems just too much to handle—you may be living with the long-term effects of a trauma—and that is PTSD.
9. If you feel bitterness or bigotry toward certain people or races—it could be the result of trauma---and subsequently of PTSD.
10. If you are convinced that everyone is against you or out to get you, you may be living with PTSD.
11. If the BIG problems of the world are a constant source of worry to you, but your own backyard is a mess—that's the result of PTSD.
12. If you are drinking too much, it could be the result of PTSD.
13. If drugs make the world an easier place to tolerate, then you could be suffering with PTSD.
14. If you are suspicious of others who did not share your experiences, that could be PTSD.
15. If you mistrust big organizations and their motivations, that feeling could be part of PTSD.
16. If you think the government is against you personally—that comes from PTSD.

17. If you have little interest in the feelings or concerns of others-even your spouse and children—that too is a result of PTSD.
18. If your continuing nightmares bring back the trauma you suffered---that's PTSD.
19. If you physically lash out at your bed partner while you dream about protecting yourself from harm— you could be reliving a trauma and be trying to protect yourself from old enemies—PTSD in one of its most insidious forms.
20. If you unwillingly relive the traumatic events of the past with frightening clarity—it is because of PTSD.
21. If you find yourself becoming overly angry, or you have a short fuse on your anger at people or situations, attribute it to PTSD.

THE DISTORDED PERCEPTION OF PTSD

The mental disturbances that result from PTSD are very disturbing not only to the person with the disorder, but to family and associates because the actions and reactions are not appropriate to the surroundings and atmosphere in which they occur.

One's life can be moving along in good order, except for the usual intermittent problems. One who has lived through a trauma can, on a clear summer day, surrounded by a happy and healthy family, have a flashback of the trauma powerful enough to shatter the pleasant and joyous mood for a day or for a week.

Individuals who have seen innocent children destroyed in war, find it hard to enjoy watching children play. The impact of seeing dead children returns when they see the joy and laughter of children having fun. The connection in their unconscious is too strong to break, i.e. children at play will be killed and their joy of living be cut short. Also children screaming while playing, or when they are hurt will cause an extreme reaction from one with PTSD. Those who live with this thought process will avoid children at play, and may be visibly upset at the normal childish merriment without really knowing why. We think this reaction is part of the need to hide from the enemy, to maintain silence in a danger area is part of the unreasonable disturbance. The necessity for refugees to hide anywhere to avoid contact with troops or police will contribute to a life time concern for silence and stillness.

Concentration camp survivors admit the feeling of responsibility for children is sometimes more than they can handle. They watched as children were separated from their parents in the camps. They felt the hopelessness of the situation and helplessness of parents to protect their child. The feeling of helplessness to aid the children in the camps, persists for years, and often interferes with loving care normal parents can give their children. The demands of their captors for order and silence under penalty of punishment is so ingrained, the reaction is without conscious thought. The displacement of place does not enter into the demand for orderly conduct, and absolute quiet.

As time goes on, the sufferer consciously avoids enjoying the pleasures of life. The fear that such enjoyable times will always be destroyed by the ever present upsetting unconscious memories dulls the ability to take pleasure in life itself.

AN OUT OF PHASE DISORDER

Post Traumatic Stress Disorder is an "out of phase" disorder. Those who suffer with PTSD can no longer identify with their peers. The sense of values they have lived with for years no longer serves them. They complain of feeling "ill at ease," because what has worked for them in the past has lost its validity. Friends, family and co-workers sense the changes, but have no idea how to help. The lack of physical complaints confuses everyone. Frustrated at the inability to handle the effects of PTSD causes the patient often rail at the big problems of society. It is much easier to voice concern at the excesses of government, than it is to face the new set of fears that cause loss of sleep, loss of libido, feelings of being all alone, separate and different from peers.

Patients often ask how they have been able to function for many years, without the intense impact Post Traumatic stress brings to them in their mid life. The explanation is a simple one. As we grow and develop, the social compact expected by society takes over without conscious effort. Psychiatry labels this process "imprinting." Our parents, teachers, and elders tell us how we are expected to act as our life progresses, even to the time of our dotage. We accept this imprinting by osmosis, with little cognitive effort. We are expected to get educated, marry, have children, start on a career path, and take on other obligations pressed on us by families, employers, the church and our community. By taking up this charge we consciously and unconsciously put the troubles of the past behind us. The requirements of our day to day life leave little time for us to stare at the past. The effects of trauma, while no longer in our consciousness are nonetheless a part of our thinking.

Once we have suffered a trauma, PTSD continues to hide itself in our unconscious. It seems to come to the fore as men and women approach what is loosely termed "middle age." At this time the demands of career, parenthood, and earlier efforts of getting established in a life have passed. This is a time for the relaxation of tensions. One now feels settled, safe and comfortable. A kind of letting down from the stresses of living comes into play. As vitality decreases, physical and psychological burdens can no longer be denied. Memories may return with reinforced strength. The symptoms of PTSD can now force their way into this peaceful scene. PTSD forces us into actions we do not understand. This unconscious process is not an excuse for anti-social behavior, but it is a major reason for some aberrant behavior. Therapy to relieve the pressures can bring understanding, and hope for relief. We can change when we can uncover, accept and attempt to modify these unconscious but powerful drives.

Father Philip Blake, S.J. says the "Noonday Devil," the seemingly diabolical phenomena that afflicts so many people, arrives in this noontime of their lives. This is a time when the shadow side of our being emerges and demands entry. Included in this change are the effects of Post Traumatic Stress Disorder. Dasberg (1987) agrees, saying "As our physical constitution declines, and mental capabilities dwindle, emptiness fills the heart, and life increasingly loses meaning."

Father Blake goes on to say that at this time in our lives we suffer the loss of the "Magic of Youth." Bewilderment replaces the permanence built over the years. The feeling of reality, once known, has disappeared. The feelings of ease and abundance, while not replaced with worry and poverty, undergo mental harassment. Memories of traumas long buried disturb the outward peace and contentment. We are psychically most vulnerable at these times of change in our lives. And these times of change are not limited to one calendar period. They occur often during one's life with no apparent pattern.

Father Blake finds other challenges that haunt those who reach this period in their life's journey:

> There is a feeling of general disillusionment. Whatever seemed to form a basis for our life no longer does. Our work, religious symbols, psychological certainty, and a particular lifestyle no longer seem adequate to the realities of life. We cannot feel, or we feel too much. We are not at home any longer with our affective life; like many other things; our feelings seem out of control. In every area of our lives, we are no longer comfortable with whatever title has previously managed to encompass our being rather well. We experience a sense of failure. Subjectively, whatever we have tried has not been good enough -- at parenting, or praying, or writing, or, especially, at loving. Ironically, others often view us as eminently successful. As we become aware of our failures in the past, our inadequacy now, and our uncertainty about the future, not only do we recognize that we have failed, but also that it is our fault. We are unsure, left to our own

devices, how to change this sad reality. We suffer from a sense of loneliness: Our struggles are our own, unique, unspeakable and unshared. We grapple with a sense of being so terribly different from everyone we have known, or even to ourselves.

We develop a last chance mentality, especially sexually, but often in other parts of life as well. I need to do it <u>now</u> or sooner, or I never will. Life is slipping away. We experience a sense of disconnectedness from ourselves, others, and especially from God. Whatever worked before in prayer or life to help make connections seems inadequate now.[1]

Depression in various degrees, and varied intensity, is always somewhat there . . . like the sadness at death, the death of ourselves, or parts of that self that we had known, and, if not loved, at least depended upon.

We now have an obsession with the past: A growing and continuing desire to understand where we have come from, our family, our religious roots, our nature and nurturing, consciously or unconsciously needing to know why we are as we are. We may make a move, trying to find something. Though we hope to discover some new life, some prince or principle of peace, we always bring ourselves with us.

During these vulnerable times, we begin to doubt our family traditions, or tribal myths. We do not yet have anything to replace them. We have accepted ideas such as:

1. We should do more than we are paid for.
2. We should not become angry.
3. Family members are obliged to understand father or mother or both.
4. If others are not like us, they are strange.
5. Everyone should get married and have children.
6. The leaders are always right (most of the time).
7. Security is the most important thing in life.
8. Don't be too happy or you will be badly disappointed.
9. Character is like a white sheet of paper, once smudged can never be clean again.
10. Your word is your bond, (but it can be re-negotiated).
11. Keep your own counsel.
12. Believe the myths told you by your parents and elders.
13. Accept that war and conflict are inevitable.
14. We have no real control over the fate that rules us.

Now we wonder if those truisms ever had any value, or will be of use in our future. They surely do not seem to have any value in our present mental state. This state of mind is explosive when combined with the residual effects of trauma.

Fortunately, there is a silver lining to trauma, as Dasberg (1987) states,

> The stress of the Holocaust has taught us that human beings can undergo extreme traumatic experiences, become deeply impaired, and yet still retain the ability to rehabilitate their ego forces. They continue to have an increased vulnerability to stress situation, but also a greater sensitivity

towards fellow humans, a greater capacity for empathy, and a greater appreciation for the higher values in life. [2]

We find agreement with this concept from Viktor Frankl who found meaning in the subhuman conditions of the Nazi concentration camps, from the writings of Carl Jung, and in the teachings of the twelve step programs.

MISDIAGNOSIS

Because those who meet with trauma try to forget the incidents, misdiagnoses continue to plague suffers of Post Traumatic Stress Disorder. Mental health practitioners with no understanding of the results of PTSD, pick out the symptoms of mental disturbance with which they are familiar. The usual diagnosis is schizophrenia. Many of the difficulties of the schizophrenic are common to one who lives with PTSD. The symptoms of narcissism, paranoia, avoidance, and selective amnesia are part of schizophrenia and of PTSD. The psychologist or doctor often fails to tie these many specifics to the complexity of Post Traumatic Stress Disorder.

Difficulties that arrive long after the event has faded from conscious memory show up in disturbed sleep; short temper; hyper alertness; avoidance of anything that could refresh memories of the trauma; a feeling that life is useless; an unwillingness to make long term commitments; often drug or alcohol abuse; nightmares; and in severe cases, poor judgment, impaired concentration and thought processes. Those who live with these symptoms, often have no idea why they feel this way. Simply stated, they were immediately infused with these feelings at the time of trauma.

PTSD causes distorted thinking in the sufferers. This result has nothing to do with intelligence, nor does it mean a mental decline. It is simply a twist in the immediate way you react to certain events or people in your life. PTSD, if not diagnosed early after the trauma occurred, may not show up in its most virulent forms for years. During that time, the victim can experience many strange or unreasonable reactions to ordinary life occurrences.

WHAT TO LOOK FOR

Fortunately, therapists who understand what happened in the past, and that trauma's effect on what is happening now can help to modify the symptomatic results of PTSD. Experiencing a trauma, and suffering from the results of that trauma, causes those who have lived through it to react in certain ways. Only an experienced therapist can uncover the hundreds of ramifications of Post Traumatic Stress Disorder. Some of these are described in the paragraphs below. If you or a loved one has PTSD, you will recognize some of them.

If persons, or groups of persons, cause you to become emotionally disturbed and physically agitated, you may be reacting to an event or series of events in your past that your conscious mind no longer recalls. This creates the "I don't know why, but I just don't like foreigners," or other broadly defined groups. It can be the basis for bigotry or other intolerant attitudes.

Post Traumatic Stress Disorder may cause a mental upset when you are in certain geographical locations, experience unusual weather, or find yourself in some types of buildings that are large and overwhelming in their sheer volume of space, or in confined quarters. These conditions can stir memories deeply buried in your unconscious. Odors, noises, textures, perceived sights, or tastes may disturb you. These attacks on your senses will be completely out of proportion to the actual conditions.

Some situations or events over which you have no control cause you great mental distress. You might find yourself greatly upset because no one in authority seems to care about the proper manner to dispose of atomic waste or take care of the environment.

You may have trouble sleeping. Your mind continues to ruminate over poorly defined social problems, or constantly ponder personal matters that cannot be immediately resolved. As a result, you find yourself awake almost all night. You may be afraid to go to sleep for the nightmares that can come.

Nightmares of the trauma return on a regular basis. You could cry out, talk in your sleep or physically attack your spouse in the sleep state. Often you will awaken in a sweat. You might have flashbacks, a powerful feeling the trauma is happening again. You experience the feeling of helplessness experienced at the time of the trauma. The terror is with you *right now; it is not a memory.* These feelings often occur during the half sleep when we are in that state of limbo when we are no longer asleep, but yet not fully awake.

The feeling might persist that others are out to get you. This can show up by constant concern that you are being cheated, or that you are not being treated fairly. You might now own a gun or guns, and other weapons. You are in a constant state of alert against what you do not know, but IT is, or THEY are out there and are trying to get you.

You refuse to watch television, go to movies, look at pictures, or read about certain places in which the trauma took place. Again, the conscious memory can be buried so deeply; you cannot determine your powerful anathema to these activities. If the subject comes up in conversation, you generally refuse to talk about it, or become greatly disturbed if you do become involved in a discussion.

You may not be able to remember major parts of the trauma. One who has been caught in a forest fire may not be able to recall the sound of forest fire, the time of day, or how they found themselves in the forest. Someone who survived an earthquake might only remember the noise and dust. Combat veterans speak of the dream like quality of battle, and often can not recall specific events.

Your ability to pursue your job and take care of your person or your surroundings may be markedly diminished. You experience a major reduction in caring about the necessary maintenance of your own life.

You can lose interest in inter-personal relations. This will be evidenced by withdrawal from other people, ranging from merely wanting to be alone much of the time, to totally withdrawing from society. These symptoms can be exacerbated by use of drugs or alcohol. At best, you will feel a detachment from others with whom you have been close.

One of the most tragic aspects of PTSD is the deterioration of loving feelings. This is most often toward parents, siblings, or spouses, but it can show itself in an unwillingness to make close contact with any human, no matter how young or innocent. In spite of this lack of capacity to feel affection, the sufferer often transfers this basic human need for contact with other living things to animals. This kind of affection allows those with PTSD to enjoy the feeling of love without any reciprocal demands. Often there is a cycle of marriage followed by divorce. Or loveless marriages continue to be held together by a mutual need for economic support.

Long range plans are continually put on hold. Those with PTSD find themselves unable to commit to any demanding future commitments. They simply drift from one day to the next. There is a feeling that the future offers nothing, or will never come.

You could be constantly angry. Sometimes you feel a low-grade dissatisfaction with everything and everybody. Often there is real hostility toward the world in general. You seethe inwardly at events and toward people with whom you come in contact, no matter how casual. Road rage is an example of this symptom. You are furious at those on the road with you because they drive a different kind of car, or do not drive in the way you expect.

You could find solace in dissociation. In dissociation you mentally leave your physical body for a less demanding place. This human trait allows us to avoid pain, either physical or mental by mentally removing our body from reality. We are unaware of the fact that our mind has gone to a less stressful place than our body occupies. This is selective amnesia when our mind chooses to forget unpleasant events or situations. Unfortunately, our unconscious continues to absorb the torment. Consciously we are more comfortable, but the unconscious mind continues to take in and store the unpleasantness around us. Meditation, a form of dissociation, is not this psychic displacement, but rather a conscious, deliberate calming exercise to find mental peace.

In the following chapters we will discuss in more detail how these symptoms have affected individuals with Post Traumatic Stress Disorder. You will see how they react, and how they have learned to accept and modify the aftermath of their traumas. In these examples you may see yourself or a loved one, and find hope to live with this baffling problem.

CHAPTER TWO

THE CHARACTERISTICS OF PTSD

Those who continue to live with the results of trauma bury the event deeply in their unconscious. They simply refuse to talk about it. A good example of this came from a group that had been in the same prison camps in Germany. They met for the first time in more than 25 years. At a gathering over coffee to reminisce about their lives in the camps, many stories were told. Most of the wives had never heard any of the stories from their husbands before. One said,"When he came home, he said, 'It's a closed chapter.' And that was the end of it. I knew nothing of his war experiences until today." One of the senior men in the Department of Veterans Affairs told me his father was a prisoner of war in World War II and he never spoke of it. Fifty years after the experience he met a group of former prisoners at a VA facility; It was like someone opened a valve under tremendous pressure. His son said after that meeting with those who had shared his trauma, his father never stopped talking about it, powerful evidence of the need to bring the old feelings to consciousness.

Part of that reticence to discuss the trauma is the personal unwillingness to reopen the wound. Memory is unreliable. We have found that many who live with PTSD have an understandable distorted memory of the event. Because it was so far beyond normal human experience, its very intensity is difficult to relate to other life experiences. The conscious mind distorts the memory, often intensifying trauma.

Before a trauma happens, there is a belief in personal invulnerability. If you feel "it can't happen to me," there is a lack of apprehension. Because there is no sense of vulnerability, you lived with total disbelief that any injury can happen to you. We also held a perception that our private world was meaningful and comprehensible. Trauma causes us to lose the earlier view of ourselves in a positive light, when we held ourselves in high self-esteem, and felt that we were worthy persons.

We come to realize that we are no longer capable of continuing in present status, i.e., athletes are no longer able to maintain their physical prowess. Professionals become too old to handle the demands of their position. Soldiers are no longer physically capable of functioning in a combat unit. The inexorable process of mental and physical capacity will continue the decline.

LOSS OF INNOCENCE

When trauma occurs the assumptions that allowed us to have a peaceful psyche are shattered. Those who now suffer from Post Traumatic Stress Disorder experienced a trauma for which they were totally unprepared. One encounters a traumatic experience with an ingenuous attitude powerful enough to cause Post Traumatic Stress Disorder. In cases of PTSD particularly in the case of civilian soldiers, the trauma of combat is intensified by at least a relative innocence of spirit. This loss of innocence is easy enough to understand when we become aware of the long term effect of trauma.

PTSD sufferers live with a feeling of being greatly damaged and that they were totally innocent of any wrong doing. In this ingenuousness, they adjust in many ways in an unconscious effort to recapture that former purity of heart. In the Stockholm syndrome, the victim allies with the enemy. This strange behavior is often found in abduction cases where the abducted person goes along with the abductor in a self-preservation attitude. That early cooperation becomes a way of life when the victim accepts the attitudes and temperament of the captor and may no longer feel victimized.

Recurrent and intrusive recollections of the event cause the sufferer to react as though experiencing the event at that moment. Because of these frightening occurrences, the person makes a deliberate effort to avoid thoughts, feelings, or conversations about the traumatic event. Spouses of people who have been involved in such a violent confrontation have been kept totally in the dark about the experience. Many refuse to discuss their experiences. Part of this reticence comes from a realization by the victim of a trauma that others simply cannot relate to the dread, fear, and fright of the occurrence. When those closest to you express disbelief in many indirect ways, it creates more of the feeling of being misunderstood. You might feel that others simply do not care about the horrifying incident or period of time. PTSD sufferers will avoid activities, situations, or people who arouse recollections of the trauma. Many war veterans refuse to join veteran's organizations.

Jorge Seprum, a Buchenwald survivor said about his experiences: "One can never tell one's son, if one has a son. One tells it best to strangers, because one is less involved." (1980 pp. 404-405) [3]. Part of that feeling is because disbelief from an outsider is less painful than from a loved one who we thought could understand, but cannot.

This avoidance of reminders will keep people away from geographical areas, or specific locations where the trauma occurred. Important dates or other data surrounding the trauma may be impossible to recall, a kind of selective amnesia.

Some force themselves to return to the scene. Others do academic research to determine the conditions in which they found themselves, and the reasons for the situation. These efforts assist in placing the trauma in a realistic frame. Therapists speak of re-framing the experience. That effort is intended to put the trauma in a fresh light in order not to see it in the fog of twisted memory. An insurance company advertisement showed the outline of a windshield with only white space inside of it. The caption said "Picture of an accident about to happen." That is a simplistic but accurate portrayal of the difficulty in remembering the details of a trauma. It is vital to become somewhat comfortable with the memories of a trauma to make it real, and make the memory accurate in order to deal with what really happened.

There is value in revisiting the scene of trauma when the psyche is ready. One soldier had nightmares about a particular place almost nightly for fifty years. After he went back to see the locale, the nightmares ended. His distorted memory was replaced with reality. The same process is turning on the lights when a child has had a bad dream to show there is nothing in its room to fear.

When one thinks of the terms used to describe trauma, the inability to create an accurate memory becomes clearer. People who have been traumatized use terms like knocked down, bowled over, flattened, smacked in the face, ambushed, and beaten down.

Once the traumatic incident is over, most people try to get on with their life by attempting to put the experience behind them. This conscious effort works for a while. But the feeling of betrayal by higher authority, government, the church, and family and even God intensifies the desire to forget the experience. The conscious effort is of little avail. The memory does fade from conscious memory, but the subconscious betrays the conscious by nurturing the effects of the trauma.

FLASHBACKS

Flashbacks are defined as a brief, clear, and intense memory of a traumatic occurrence. The person experiencing a flashback feels as though the incident is happening again. Fortunately flashbacks while extremely frightening are of short duration, lasting only seconds. The impact, including physiological damage, remains.

Flashbacks come at strange times. One would think the caring atmosphere of a well reputed hospital would be the last place for a frightening flashback to happen. A friend who was spent three years in a concentration camp needed some surgery. On the appointed date, he reported to the hospital waiting room with a number of other patients. An attendant led them into a large room with beds on each of the four walls. Reading from a clipboard, she announced "When your name is called, go to the bed with the number I call out, close the drapes, take off all of your clothes and put them in the bag on the bed, put on a hospital gown and sit down on the bed. Then wait until your number is called."

He immediately felt he was back in a camp. His personal identity was gone, replaced by a number. He went on to say, "All of the familiar trappings that gave me individuality were now in a plastic bag that would be disposed of by persons unknown to me. When my number was called from a list on a clipboard, the stress of roll call in the camps returned with great intensity. I was in effect, naked and helpless. My personal possessions were taken from me, just as they had been in the Gulag. No longer was I an individual, but rather a number. I was to be moved to a strange and frightening place, like the gas chambers. The terror was almost overwhelming. The memory bothers me to this day. I think it was more intense because I thought I was in a place of protection and safety when it happened. I did not expect that wave of abhorrent memory."

Michelene Maurel, a French woman who survived a German concentration camp, tells about how well entrenched the memory is in the mind of the returnee in her book, *An Ordinary Camp.*

> Each survivor has brought his camp back with him; he tries to obliterate it; he tries to stifle in the barbed wire and under the straw mattresses all those despairing schmustics, but suddenly a date or a photograph brings back the entire camp around him. But the entire camp rises again slowly, for it has not been destroyed and nothing has made up for a single day of suffering. (1958, p. 141).[4]

UNWILLINGNESS TO THINK ABOUT OR DISCUSS THE TRAUMA

Many who have lived through a trauma refuse to discuss it with anyone, including those closest to them, such as their spouse or other members of the family. The pain of the memory is more than the victim is willing to relive. We know that talking about the trauma and the attendant feelings that it created, is the best therapy. A trauma creates a melange of feelings that are difficult to sort out alone. Good therapy puts the trauma in a perspective the individual can understand and accept. Denial that the trauma affected the survivor is common. Part of that attitude comes from the "be strong" training of young men, and the strength women are expected to show to their family. The actions and reactions show the deep seated effect the particular shock created, and continues to plague one who suffered a trauma.

The daughter of a survivor of the Titanic sinking, said her mother never would speak of the disaster. We can only imagine the terror created when that great ship, which offered such comfort and safety, disappeared into the sea. The loss experienced by those men and women, was not simply the sinking of a great ship, but the loss of their home, their possessions, and their loved ones. Their core sense of worldly security destroyed. For some, the conscious memory became too distressing to recall.

Historians have said that part of the intensity of the Titanic disaster, was a loss of innocence. The realization came to the passengers and later to the whole world that no matter how great are the accomplishments of man, there are more powerful forces that can destroy them. In the early 1900's the world was living in the prosperity of the Industrial Revolution. In manufacturing, agriculture, and trade, the world economy was prospering. The passenger list of the Titanic carried the names of many of the world's wealthiest and most powerful people. The world was at the feet of these leaders of industry and finance. One can only imagine the attitude of omnipotence they may have felt.

Position, wealth and power meant nothing to those in the lifeboats. Instead they now faced confusion and bewilderment at what was happening to them. Certainly they must have wondered why they were being subjected to this terrible calamity. Nothing they had done should have put them into this distressing situation. They had followed all the rules they knew to become passengers on the ship. No overt action on their part contributed to the disaster. With no culpability, they were now in an uncontrollable, frightening situation. In their minds they had to be screaming out "Why me, God?"

Survivors can put the conscious memory behind themselves, by refusing to discuss the trauma with anyone. But the impact on the unconscious cannot be erased. Fearful and possible subsequent angry reactions, one of the results of Post Traumatic Stress Disorder will continue to plague the survivor of any trauma. An obvious conscious reaction to surviving a ship sinking would be to avoid any further travel by sea. But less obvious or overt reactions will result. In the case of a survivor of the Titanic sinking, being alone in the darkness could be an unresolved fear. Separation anxiety had to be maximized when the ship, its crew, the waiters and stewards who had made the first part of the trip safe and comfortable, all were gone. There was no help available. The terrible loneliness of the vast open sea, cut off from all that offered succor, was an overpowering and terrifying experience.

The effect on survivors of a trauma can be quite different. A Mr. Lightolier, the first officer of the Titanic and the only officer who survived the sinking is credited with saving many lives. Because of his capability and dedication to the safety of the passengers entrusted to him, he was truly a hero in the tragic drama of the Titanic sinking. He stayed with the ship until in his words, "the ship left me, I did not leave the ship." He had stepped into the water as the deck slid under the surface. His training as a seaman and many years at sea no doubt had prepared him for the dangers of ocean travel. While the loss of a ship as grand as the Titanic surely caused him pain, he was well aware of the hazards of the sea. Once he was able to appraise what he had done to minimize the loss of life, he may well have been satisfied that he had done his duty. The probability of PTSD in one as experienced as Lightolier is minimal. We found this same dichotomy between the professional soldier and the draftee. The best trained men came through combat with the least residual mental anguish.

DISTORTED MEMORY

Memory of trauma is usually inaccurate. Part of that difficulty is the selective amnesia in PTSD. Another is trying to look back at such a bad experience analytically. One major problem is judgment is now improved by life experience. Second guessing oneself is common but useless. Until the memory is brought back without distortion and examined in that light, the sufferer will be looking at the past through a clouded mirror.

One client who served two terms in Viet Nam told us in a therapy group that he knew what he had done to other humans while in combat. He had taken dozens of pictures and brought them home. He was most regretful for what he had done in the heat of battle. He was able to recognize his deeds without distortion. His deep regret and heart felt remorse were for real acts, not distorted memories. He realized he was judging the actions of a teen aged boy with the wisdom of a fifty year old man.

Hesitancy comes from fears that the story is so far beyond the listener's experience that it is incomprehensible, and unbelievable. This is why it is important to discuss the trauma and its resultant problems with qualified therapists. We say qualified, not simply educated and licensed, but those therapists who truly understand PTSD.

I DON'T REALLY CARE ABOUT ANYONE

A lack of loving feelings, that is the inability to love another human is probably the most tragic result of Post Traumatic Stress Disorder. We think this lack is directly related to another quality of the disorder, the unwillingness to look ahead to a pleasant future. Loving needs constancy and hope. Those who cannot look to the future are unable to feel this devotion to another. We also consider this lack of loving ability as a result of the loss of innocence. Cynicism, distrust, and doubt are some of the attitudes that result from

PTSD. Those traits will undermine even the most dedicated lovers.

In war veterans particularly, we have found a continuing inability to bond with another. Multiple relationships are common. Separation and divorce is almost endemic. This inability also contributes to estrangement with children. If a child or other loved one dies or is killed it is easy to understand this unwillingness to face the possibility of the pain of loss again.

LIVING WITH HYPERALERTNESS

Another major characteristic of PTSD is an abnormal startle response. Some of this results from the withdrawal by the person with PTSD. Withdrawal seems to be the direct result of the traumatic experience. The unconscious sets up an ultra sensitive warning system in an effort, even though unnecessary, to avoid a recurrence of the trauma. Any quick movement or noise sets off this mental alarm. The fear comes back in the unconscious and then to the conscious mind, causing a sometimes violent, but always powerful reaction. In the worst cases, the patient may lash out physically at the one who created the disturbance.

ALONENESS, AVOIDANCE AND NIGHTMARES

Those who have trouble sleeping at night because they can't stop the unformed fear may be suffering with PTSD. There is a universal fear of the dark. As children we all had a bad dream or two. When we mature, the fear of darkness disappears, and a bad dream is just that. For those who live with PTSD these benign but annoying areas of the night take on a different face. There is a barrage of emotions, some of which result in sheer terror.

Everyone has an occasional nightmare. It is a perfectly normal experience, even though an uncomfortable one. Two of the most common involve falling from a great height, or of being in a huge dark space. Dream researchers attribute these almost universal bad dreams to early experiences. We are trained to fear falling by our parents or caretakers when we are very young. The admonition "Be careful, don't fall" is almost ubiquitous among parents. This kind of imprinting will probably never leave us. When the imprinted command is combined with the desire of little children to please their parents, we create a built in nightmare subject.

The fear that comes in the nightmare about huge dark space is attributed to memories of being in the womb. The terror comes from the impression of floating, combined with a total lack of control. While the genesis of both of these common nightmares is harmless enough, the continuing feelings from these early powerful impressions can disturb our sleep.

Those who live with the effects of trauma suffer recurring nightmares. We mentioned in another chapter, the recurring nightmare of a soldier about a house he entered during a time of a fierce ground battle. The nightmare was certainly not of being in the house, as he remembered that part of the experience with pleasure. The trauma resulted from the many emotions of combat mixed in with his one clear memory of the time. His dream was a sublimation of the juxtaposition of potent memories of home, and the mixture of death, dirt, and fear of armed combat. He could not consciously separate his memories of the pleasant house from the wretchedness of combat conditions. The memory of what should have been an agreeable incident instead caused him great distress and almost nightly disturbing dreams of visiting the house.

The nightmares of those who live with the after affects of trauma are from a quite a different source. The kinds of fear generated by trauma are often non-specific. That is to say the fear is potent but the ways that fear is shows up may have no relation to the original trauma. We can easily understand that one who lived through an airplane crash would not want to fly again, or would do so with great trepidation. However, that specific fear can expand to other kinds of transportation, which will cause all sorts of interpersonal problems that appear not to have any connection with the airplane disaster.

One client, a war veteran, awakens in a panic from the dream of lying helpless on a battlefield. The cognizant reality of being awake in his home continues to be overpowered by a feeling of raw terror. He has no conscious memory of the fear he felt while he lay wounded and exposed in the aftermath of a fire fight. He was unable to protect himself for the time he lay there because of the nature of his wounds. The strong unconscious memory of the need for protection at that time now keeps him awake with a loaded gun in his hand until dawn.

Another man who served two years in Viet Nam has recurring nightmares of in his words, "a backyard full of black pajamas (North Viet Nam soldiers)." He awakens with feelings of panic, often perspiring through his night clothes. The dream is so real, he has to get out of bed, turn on the flood lights, and tour his back yard before he can go back to sleep. Even though he is consciously aware that he has had "the nightmare", he cannot go back to sleep until he has followed this ritualistic checking of his property. He told us, "I know there is nothing there, but I cannot help myself. I have to check it out."

Much of our work has been with men and women who served in the military. Most traumas occurred in combat situations or war time conditions. The obvious stress that condition causes is obvious. Some PTSD resulted from training accidents. Do not think that the military establishment has a corner on the creation of Post Traumatic Stress. We have found it in many clients who have never been near the military. The sources are many, and in some cases, seemingly harmless at the time they occurred.

An experience as apparently innocuous as the course of instruction leading to advanced college degrees can be extremely traumatic and cause post trauma nightmares. One client who was graduated with high honors continues to experience nightmares that involve rejection from non-specific groups or individuals. She discussed with us the strain she endured while working toward her Masters degree and later her Doctorate. She lived in constant fear that she would not be able to complete her work to the satisfaction of her mentors. In spite of the fact that today she is an extremely well regarded member of her profession, the dreams of failure and rejection continue to haunt her. Not even a physical review of her diplomas, licenses and commendations on the wall of her office offset this potent remaining result of her earlier educational traumas.

One of our clients is a dog breeder. She has enjoyed a long and close relationship with her dogs. She was attacked by one of the dogs she had raised from a puppy. The attack was unprovoked and vicious. The flesh in her fore and upper right arm was badly torn, one forearm bone was bitten through, and another was seriously bruised. After many years, the wound has not totally healed, and even though the arm is again usable, it has never returned to the flexibility and strength she had previously.

She has a recurring nightmare that begins with her dreaming she has awaken to discover her right arm is missing. She gets out of bed and looks out the window into the swimming pool area. The dog that attacked her is running clockwise around the pool with her arm in his mouth. When she tries to get to the dog, he reverses his direction. She is unable to catch him, or to get him to stop. Finally, the dog drops the arm into the pool. She awakens in a panic feeling for her arm.

That kind of dream in view of the trauma that started it is easy to understand. But the feelings that this client lives with in other areas of her life are somewhat removed from this straight forward attack and recovery incident. She finds herself much more suspicious of people, a feeling that arose from the violation of her trust by her dog. She also lives with a feeling of aloneness and loneliness which formerly was filled by the company of her dogs. She thinks she has lost some her nurturing capacity with living things, including other humans, again because of the attack by one in whom she had great trust. No longer does she feel comfortable in the association with large animals, not necessarily dogs. This is the hyper alertness caused by PTSD, and the loss of innocence we find in so many with PTSD.

NARCISSISM & EGOCENTRICITY

Narcissism and egocentricity are common features of Post Traumatic Stress Disorder. When we consider the intensity of traumatic incidents, and the concern for survival that are part of them, narcissism, and self centeredness, the concern with self is an understandable result. These personalities characteristics create great problems in interpersonal relationships.

SUSPICION

Those who live with PTSD are suspicious people. We equate their suspicion with the destruction of innocence caused by trauma. Prior to a traumatic event, there is that feeling of invincibility. Our world is regulated and understandable. We accept that there are regulations with which most live, that there are governmental and private organizations that maintain order, and will rescue us from danger. After a traumatic event, the previous belief that we would be protected by this established order is fractured. The result is a continuing disbelief in the omnipotence of our social order. Institutions in which we believed become suspect.

"NOBODY REALLY UNDERSTANDS ME"

Viktor Frankl wrote "Those who were there (in concentration camps) will understand what we endured. Those who were not there will never understand." [5]

For those who served in Viet Nam, the rest of the world was "out there" and they had no real connection with it. A common statement was "For a while after I came home, I tried to explain what it was like, but I finally gave up." Most any one who suffers from PTSD comes to the realization that any attempt to make others understand the effect of the trauma is a useless effort. This is not to demean the willingness to understand and help by those who have concern and sympathy. It is clearly a case of not being able to comprehend the depth of feelings those who endure PTSD live with. The fear resulting from a natural disaster, the loss of a home by fire, or the agony of a vehicle accident is and impossible experience to relate to another. Even those who have suffered similar accidents have a difficult time relating. An exception is those who have lived through the same disaster. An unusual immediate bonding occurs with those who suffered a common catastrophe.

PEOPLE ARE NO DARN GOOD

To one who has experienced a trauma, a feeling of being apart or disturbing loneliness often results. The inability to relate the experience to others and the resulting anguish creates a barrier that is difficult or impossible to cross. The human psyche does not like rejection. The perceived lack of interest in the traumatic event is looked upon as rejection, or disbelief. The natural reaction is to withdraw. We found that part of the disorder was the feeling of rejection that turned into a defense mechanism of deciding that all people were foes. Those with PTSD became loners, and the resultant lack of confidants or friends contributed to the cycle of loneliness and being apart from society. Suppressed fears that came out as anger further contributes to isolation.

WHAT'S THE USE OF TRYING?

The shattering of innocence that accompanies trauma contributes to a powerful feeling of apathy toward living. Apathy is a survival mode. Viktor Frankl identified apathy as a common defense mechanism in concentration camp inmates and prisoners of war. This mechanism can come into play with debilitating effects in life after incarceration. This is not day dreaming, but rather a general mental malaise that can cause great difficulty in the normal functions of daily living. The major characteristic of apathy is a negative attitude toward the future. And a disinterest in what is happening presently.

Another aspect of handling the memory of trauma is to take the attitude "It didn't mean nothin'," a common attitude to avoid discussing the situation with an outsider.

When the attitude of a loner is combined with the suspicion that people not only do not understand, but do not care, an attitude that it "Wasn't much, or wasn't so bad" results. Eric Williams, an English soldier who became a prisoner of war described it this way when asked "What was it like?"

> It wasn't so bad in some ways. But, he wondered as he answered how he could describe the damp barracks blocks . . . the dirty and bearded kriegies queued up for midday ration of cabbage water. . describe the crowd of lonely figures, lonely in spite of a thousand like them. Of starvation rations . . . (p. 254). [6]

I CAN'T SEEM TO FORGET IT

The power of memory in dealing with trauma is easy to understand. We all have said, "I'm glad it didn't happen to me (or anyone really close to me.) That someone carries a conscious and disturbing memory of a trauma is understandable. Anniversary dates are particularly hard on those who live with PTSD. One client of ours refused to leave his house on the anniversary date of his horrible accident. The conscious memory causes enough problems. The unconscious is a real wrongdoer. It never forgets. On an anniversary date long forgotten, uneasiness and annoyance can plague those who live with this insidious disorder.

STRANGE BEHAVIOR PATTERNS

"I know I am different, but I don't know why, or what to do about it." This is a common feeling expressed by those who live with the results of trauma. Reactions to people and places are more intense. Reactions to situations cause vehement actions that do not fit the circumstances. Our clients find it difficult to understand why everyone does not share their depth of concern. Those who have lived through natural disasters are constantly on the alert for signs of another catastrophe. They are disturbed over what they perceive as a lackadaisical attitude toward emergency preparation. People who have lived with shortages go to great lengths to avoid privation, and cannot understand why others do not share their anxiety. This seeming lack of interest in self-preservation efforts can cause even more distress. The actions of someone with PTSD seem logical. It is the rest of the world that is out of sync.

ARRESTED DEVELOPMENT

Intense trauma can cause an arrest of development. The emotional reaction to a current situation is perceived by the unconscious mind as the original trauma, so the effect will be the same as those experienced during the original trauma. Thus a middle-aged person will react as a teenager, or even as a young child. This arrested development can arise in other actions of the victim. His or her interpersonal relations are often out of phase for their calendar age and presumed state of maturity. Because the victim does not react to all life situations in an age appropriate manner, chaos results, particularly with those closest to the sufferer.

Certainly if the victim is stuck, the normal moral development as analyzed by Kohlberg stops. This failure to develop morally creates the teen age mentality in a middle aged person. They cannot get unstuck. Their capacity to develop normally was removed by trauma. To learn and accept the moral codes and rules of conduct is a challenging task, often ignored to the dismay of the family and friends of the injured party.

OTHER CAUSES OF PTSD

We know that PTSD is the result of many kinds of traumas. In conversation with our friends, we have all discussed the effects that an auto accident, a drowning, house fire, earthquake, or other natural disaster has had on people we know or have read about.

We discovered that many retired professional athletes suffer from Post Traumatic Stress Disorder. The loss of physical strength or injury, age and the lack of continuing recognition by the fans bring on PTSD. Most important and often overlooked by counselors and therapists is the loss of the endorphin rush created by intensive training, and the raw enjoyment of the combat of the game. The trauma in these cases was not the result of an instantaneous event, but rather an accumulation over a long period of time. When the excitement generated by intensive training and the games are over, the energy supplied by the natural creation of endorphins in the brain and the attendant high it produced was gone. We think the realization that the game was over for life, and that the quiet of retirement, forced or not, caused great mental bewilderment.

The same problem faced by the professional athlete exists in the person who has been in a combat situation for a long time. He or she begins to enjoy the endorphin rush. Even though the reaction is to danger and destruction, the feeling afterwards is one of great satisfaction the result of their body's creation of natural chemicals offsetting the intense physical and emotional demands of combat. In a strange way, those who have lived through combat miss the excitement, and the rush of endorphins.

The endorphin rush comes from the fright-flight, or fight syndrome. When our cave man ancestors were faced with danger, their hearts began to beat faster by their body's creation of adrenaline, which in turn caused their breathing to increase, and their concentration to become more keen. An additional factor is the body force which created the endorphins, which are one of the neuropeptides.

The neuropeptides perform various functions in the body including the secretion of endorphins. Endorphins affect emotion and offset pain. When we watch a runner, or a game player, they are generating endorphins to offset the pain and weariness they feel as the result of their physical effort. Just as one would become addicted to a drug, athletes become addicted to the adrenaline and resulting endorphin rush. Once the super effort is finished, the body returns to its normal processes. The action was invigorating including the pleasure of the endorphins that were generated.

The need for this physical capability and mental stimulation in antiquity was a reasonable one. It was necessary to speed up the body to fight the saber toothed tiger or the mammoth. In our modern society we do not have wild animals to kill for survival, so the need for the internally generated rush is not necessary. However, endorphins are an addicting internal pleasure-inducing chemical. The desire to recreate those feelings of excitement continues. The dissatisfaction with a peaceful life is common. This is the PTSD not from living through an immediate trauma, but it creates the same living problems for the retired athlete as it does for the retired military person.

The effect of armed combat on men was well described by Ernie Pyle, the famed World War II correspondent.who wrote of them:

> A soldier who has been a long time in the line does have a 'look' in his eyes that anyone who knows about it can discern. It's a look of dullness, eyes that look without seeing, eyes that see without conveying any image to the mind . . . (A

look of) exhaustion, lack of sleep, tension for too long, wariness that is too great, fear beyond fear, misery to the point of numbness, a look of surpassing indifference to anything anyone can do. It's a look I dread to see on men. [7]

Is it any wonder the experience not only comes home with such men, but that it stays in their unconscious forever?

ELIZABETH

Elizabeth loved animals, especially her dogs. She showed them in many arenas. Three of her Rottweilers were champions. After her older dogs died, she found a Rottweiller puppy about two months old. When the dog was grown, about two years old, he attacked her without warning. He bit through the bones in her forearm, and tore the flesh in her upper arm badly. Emergency surgery to repair the damage was followed by a series of orthopedic procedures, and physical therapy to strengthen the bones and repair the flesh wounds. The processes took place over a five or six year period.

Elizabeth's former love of animals is gone. She is terrified when confronted by large dogs. She will cross the street to avoid them, even if they are leashed. She has a recurring dream of being attacked by animals, not necessarily dogs. When those dreams come, she awakens in a state of panic, and usually cannot get back to sleep.

DREAMS AND NIGHTMARES

Two of the most disturbing elements of Post Traumatic Stress Disorder are persistent nightmares and flashbacks. Flashbacks create the feeling that the event is happening again, and right now, with all of its intensity. These intrusive and disturbing memories come at unexpected times. Often they occur when everything else in one's life is in good order, making the impact of these alarming recollections is most disturbing. Nightmares happen in the innocence of sleep. Flashbacks come at a peaceful time when awake. The shattering of innocence is a sharp painful reminder of a terrible time in the past. While the time elapsed for this intrusive memory is short. The time of the results is not.

Recurring unpleasant dreams or nightmares come with sleep. To avoid the agony and terror that they bring, those with PTSD avoid sleep. Many clients have told us their bad dreams came less often as years passed, but when they did return the intensity had not dimmed. A common description is the repeat of the beginning of a nightmare usually accompanied by the feeling that the dreamer has no control in the situation. He may know what terrifying incident is about to come, but cannot stop the rerun of his nightmare. The trauma returns not in a clear well defined manner, but rather accompanied by new distortions of memory. Almost always they describe the feeling of helplessness to stop the action, no doubt a replay of the "Oh, no" reaction to the trauma. Often the dream is powerful enough for the dreamer to lash out as his bed partner, sit up in panic, and always results in a cold sweat from the reality of the memory.

Little wonder those with PTSD tolerate the misery of sleeplessness to avoid the mental punishment of their dreams.

Sleep patterns are irregular. This factor relates to hyper-alertness, another trait of PTSD. Some sufferers take unusual steps to sleep more calmly. A common one is to sleep with a weapon under the pillow or nearby. Self medication is not unusual, either alcohol, or drugs. Some men have told us they are never more than an arm's length away from a weapon anywhere in their homes.

We can attribute this part of Post Traumatic Stress Disorder to the intense fear that an event generates, together with the feelings of helplessness that accompany the fright. That lack of control equated with the total release of sleep will create the inability to sleep comfortably. There is also the very real concern that sleep will bring the nightmares.

"LEAVE ME ALONE!"

Another characteristic of PTSD is that you may wish everyone would go away and let you alone--but you are afraid of being alone. We have seen many men who isolate for no apparent reason. Their wives tell us how "he stays in his workshop—or works on his computer, and doesn't spend time with me or the kids." Everyone needs time to be alone. One writer recommended that married couples make a sign saying "Do not disturb-batteries recharging" to hang around their neck when they wanted to be alone. Certainly a non-threatening manner to be alone with their individual thoughts.

That is not what we see in those with PTSD. The poor souls live with their own particular demons, those that make them afraid to get close to someone else, or endure the agonies of paranoia. This powerful emotion comes from losing friends in a catastrophe. They feel the helplessness of seeing a dear one drown, get hit by a car, or killed in some other situation. Ill defined fears of the unknown, of the tormenting demons that grew from old forgotten terrors that persist only in whispers of the past, or events lost in the fogs of memory. All that comes through are the powerful, indefinable and deeply disturbing feelings.

It is much simpler to stay away from any relationship that can cause more pain. Changing jobs or residences is a way to avoid meaningful connection with others whose loss could bring the pain to the fore again. The immediate upset and change is preferable to the disturbance created by a possible loss of a friend.

Isolation brings another dilemma. This is typical of the problems caused by PTSD. Each ramification of the disorder is tied to another difficulty. We found that one good way to relieve the internal distress of PTSD is to talk about it with others. This can be a professional, or with someone who has lived through the same kind of trauma. Meetings of war veterans, former prisoners of war, rape victims, and other groups with members of similar backgrounds serve this function very well. Mainly we think it is the discovery by the members of the group that they are not alone in their feelings and living problems. Alcoholics Anonymous, the original 12 step group, offers not a program to stop drinking, but rather a set of rules and methods to live one day at a time. Its members help each other by mutual encouragement engendered by their common problems and experiences. One of the major benefits of group therapy is breaking the isolation element in

PTSD. One former prisoner of war told us "During withdrawal to save ourselves, we built a protection in loneliness that remained with us. Our loneliness became a way of life." (personal files.)

AVOIDANCE

Related to, but not quite the same as isolation, is the avoidance of facing the trauma head on. We have had clients tell us of not being able to go back to a place of trauma for years after the event. One man, who had lost both legs in a motorcycle accident, avoided the major street on which it had happened for three years. To avoid the area required he go a long way around. Finally, he was able to drive by, rapidly at first, and avoid the former time consuming and circuitous route. At the end, he was able to get out of his car and examine the area closely. Not until then, was he at peace with the place of his trauma. Nothing had changed except his attitude, and his return to reality.

Another client who had spent months in front line combat in Viet Nam sublimated his fears of returning to Southeast Asia by collecting coins and bills from the area. He became a recognized expert in the field. In time, he became so interested in the medium; he went back to Viet Nam to increase his knowledge and collection. The return to his place of trauma was subjugated to his interest in a totally different phase of the country. He was able to realize that life in Viet Nam, as with him, had moved on. No longer was it a place of death and dying. While the wounds of his war remain with him, he no longer has the violent reaction to anything that reminded him of his months of pain and misery.

We have worked with men who flew many combat missions in wartime. They vowed when they finished their last mission that they would never get into an airplane again. This condition is the result of continuing trauma. When one of these people has lived through the terror of being in air combat many times, the resulting relief at staying alive shows up in a refusal to take on any more risk in the air. This attitude persists in spite of cognitive acceptance of the airline's safety record.

We all know of people who will not fly, or of those afraid of being on the water, of heights, or enclosed or open places. These phobias are usually the result of many forces in a person's life. They may be the result of forgotten childhood traumas or expressed fears by parents. PTSD is a different animal. It is the result of something that happened to the individual, leaving an indelible impression, the results of which continue to plague the sufferer. With therapy, most of these phobias can be eliminated or diminished. So can the results of trauma that results in PTSD.

LEARNED HELPLESSNESS

Learned helplessness and the subsequent depression, was first mentioned by Doctor Viktor Frankl. Frankl was a prime candidate for PTSD as the result of his 44 months in a German concentration camp. Frankl was a medical doctor, but he spent all of his time in captivity at hard labor. His teachings appeared first in his classic book "Man's Search For Meaning" printed first in 1947, Frankl wrote:

> Any attempt at fighting the psycho-pathological influence on the prisoner by

> psychotherapeutic or psychohygienitic methods had to aim at giving him strength by pointing out to him a future goal to which he could look forward. . . . It is a peculiarity of man that he can only live by looking to the future. . . . And this is his salvation in the most difficult moments of his existence.

He went on to describe his technique to rise above his thinking of "the endless little problems of our miserable life . . ." He forced himself to look to the future by "observing the sufferings of the moment as though they were already in the past." (pp73-74).[5]

We have found in many whom live with PTSD, a well developed sense of helplessness and hopelessness. They are major symptoms of the disorder.

To eliminate this feeling of helplessness, one must look to the future as recommended by Dr. Frankl. The feelings of helplessness, combined with the sense of a foreshortened future, are a deadly mental combination. Most have an extremely difficult time in getting away from the learned helplessness and the attendant depression. Many who live with PTSD allow themselves to go to a continuing "pity party" often by finding groups of people who share their feelings. Instead of the self help spirit of the Twelve Step groups, which work at getting people out of the helpless and hopelessness of their addiction, in some groups often a "poor me" is the only attitude that prevails.

It is incumbent on the therapist and the family to help the sufferer to see the uselessness of continuing self pity. They must continue in their efforts to get the patient to see their future in a positive light. This is more important, when there are physical problems, which may have resulted from the original trauma that is now Post Traumatic Stress Disorder.

Places of trauma are easy to identify. Much more difficult is the resulting torment when circumstances upset the psyche. Clients have told us they do not know why certain people, places or things cause them mental distress. The results of trauma are so deeply buried that even with therapy the reasons are difficult to uncover. Many clients speak of times when they are uncomfortable in certain places. They do not know why. One of the most mysterious was a man who had lived through a particularly difficult period in his life in the Christmas season. He was able to determine consciously why the memories disturbed him at that holiday time. It was the unconscious that bothered him most. He could not accept that he was so uncomfortable in spite of his acceptance of the effects of the unfortunate time he had lived through. Because of his open questioning of his feelings, he was able to realize it was the dimmed December late afternoon sun light that took him back to the most distressing time in his travail. Interestingly, the realization has not changed his feelings about the season, but he knows why he is unhappy, and is working at changing his attitude.

Some people refuse to go back either physically or vicariously. They refuse to watch motion pictures that have anything to do with their unpleasant memories. They will not read about the locale. They refuse to deal in any way with people who remind them of their time of trauma. Their thought is by avoiding any conscious contact; the unpleasant memory will be minimized. From a conscious standpoint, that is true. It is like the pain of pushing on a sore tooth. But not pushing on the tooth does not cure the underlying abscess. It is necessary—even vital—to revisit the physical place, and endure the psychological effects including the emotions of the trauma in order to diminish the effect it holds on our life.

WHAT CAUSES THE UPSET?

This problem is one of the mysteries of PTSD. The sufferer is going along with apparent equanimity when something triggers an upset.

Anniversary dates cause deep psychic difficulties with those who have suffered trauma. The conscious memory might be able to deal with it by dismissing the problem as "history." It often happens that the date is not consciously remembered. The unconscious effect of the trauma is another story entirely. Beginning some time before the actual date you may find yourself ill at ease, short with friends and family, having difficulty sleeping, drinking or smoking more. There may be an effort to neutralize the feelings of inadequacy, by making purchases, or taking a trip that in reality is unnecessary. If one is addicted, the addiction will increase in intensity. These are all efforts of the unconscious to offset the knowledge of the impending tragedy. Remember the subconscious has no capacity to deal with time or place. It sends powerful signals the past will be repeated. It lives in the now, so the feelings are felt most powerfully.

The feeling impending doom is not imaginary as far as the psyche is concerned. It is preparing to combat the trauma again. Do not look around to find comfort in the outer world. Only by understanding where the feeling is coming from, it's true source, will the effects be modified. The effects will be lessened, but the memory will remain. The unconscious never forgets.

WHAT WILL PTSD DO TO ME?

The traumatic effects of the stressor that eventually show up in Post Traumatic Stress Disorder are intense. PTSD is presumed when there is an excessive reaction to an event that is not extreme in its character. To war veterans we say they react in a combat method to a non-combat situation. Those with PTSD may have a violent reaction when someone cuts into a waiting line; refuses to give way on the highway, or any other minor frustration that others would merely shrug off as an example of bad manners. The present day concern with rage reactions may be a ramification of early trauma.

Organizations such as the Department of Veterans Affairs, private insurance companies, state workmen's compensation departments, or the Social Security Administration have strict structures to determine if those who are applying for benefits do in fact suffer from PTSD, just as they do for any other disabling condition. One does not have to suffer from the structured pattern these organizations or insurance companies would require in order to live with the distress of PTSD. Flashbacks, nightmares, interpersonal difficulties, and/or drug and alcohol abuse may arise from an earlier trauma. The symptoms may not qualify for compensation by a government agency or private insurance company. The usual determinant factors for PTSD include significant distress or impairment in social, occupational and other areas of interpersonal functioning.

PTSD in other than its most debilitating form is often ignored. It is like hypertension, which shows few symptoms until the heart is overloaded. Because of this "lay in the weeds" characteristic, the client is thought to be fully functional until there is a reaction to a stimulus. The difficulty is in relating the reaction to a cause that is long buried. Former prisoners of war and concentration camp victims tell of buying extra food and hoarding it with no reasonable explanation. Women who have been abused as children refuse to wear revealing or even feminine styled clothing. They may not wear makeup. Those who have been in shipwrecks refuse to go near water.

There is a strong feeling that family, associates, and the medical and psychiatric professions misunderstand you. Someone said in order to empathize with one who has suffered a trauma you must get involved. Most people will not make this sacrifice. It was evident in survivors of the Holocaust, where in some cases, their Rabbi refused to discuss the concentration camp experiences of his synagogue members. (Miller 1990).[8]

Des Pres describes the survivor of trauma as

> . . . a disturber of the peace. He is a runner of the blockade, erected against the knowledge of "unspeakable" happenings. About these he undermines, without intending to, the validity of existing norms. (1976, pp. 42-43.)[9]

It has been suggested that the reason for this lack of empathy, or willingness to listen and attempt understanding is that those who have not suffered the same trauma feel an embarrassment for their wholeness. Those who have lived through such traumatic experiences become a threat without trying.

PTSD sufferers live with constant hyper alertness in day to day situations. Hyper alertness is attributed to the need to be vigilant in a combat zone, any competitive activity, or other perceived confrontive circumstance. In non- adversarial situations hyper-alertness causes unreasonable responses to unspoken messages given off by individuals. Hyper alertness causes trouble with people and places. The feeling is that everyone is trying to cheat you, whether of money, time, or ideas. Constant living with this mental tension can lead to depression, and physical exhaustion.

You may refuse to accept personal responsibility that you had a part in the trauma. Not everyone has been a party to or played a part in the trauma they suffered, but one has to look inside to accept the fact that you may have contributed to what happened. This has been expressed by prisoners of war, who feel they could have done more before being captured. We found this feeling in many veterans of the Viet Nam war, who felt they did not personally make a great enough effort, even if they suffered great physical wounds.

Charles Whiting, an English historical writer shows a keen insight into the soldier's mind in his controversial book, Ardennes, The Secret War:

> A battle does not end when the echoes of the last shots have died away. For some it means tortured nightmares. For others the permanent souring of the personality with

that eternal, overwhelming question being raised time and time again "Where did I go wrong?" (1984, p.127.) [10]

While Whiting was writing about soldiers, the same can be applied to any traumatic experience. We see it in those who have survived natural disasters, and disasters of all kinds. Many clients ask the same question "What did I do to have this happen to me?"

PTSD creates an extreme egocentric attitude. Because of the personal attack, physical or mental, a deep concern about "What is happening to me?" results. Again, you might feel that no one cares or is interested in understanding what happened, or the accompanying mental agony.

"JUST HOW MUCH CAN PTSD AFFECT MY LIFE?"

Take this self-test to see just how much PTSD can affect your life.

Answer yes or no to the statement. Use your first reaction, do not think about it too much, and don't go back to change your answer.

1. I feel misunderstood by my family and friends. YES NO
2. I often have trouble sleeping all of the night. YES NO
3. I have trouble going to sleep. YES NO
4. I often have nightmares. YES NO
5. I wish I had a gun or two available. YES NO
6, I have trouble being tender and loving. YES NO
7. I think people are generally dishonest. YES NO
8. I've had more than 3 jobs in the past 5 years. YES NO

9. I do not trust the government. YES   NO
10. I don't think people realize the problems in the country. YES   NO
11. I don' think people are very patriotic. YES   NO
12. I think society owes me a better life. YES   NO
13. I don't think people really care about me. YES NO
14. I am somewhat angry most of the time. YES   NO
15. I cannot forget the trauma I suffered. YES   NO
16. I want help to have more peace of mind. YES NO
17. I use alcohol or drugs. YES   NO
18. I have few friends. YES NO
19. I am a very social person. YES NO
20. I belong to a number of organizations. YES   NO
21. I am willing to go back to where my trauma happened. YES NO
22. I think another trauma just as bad can happen again. YES   NO
23. I feel mature. YES   NO
24. I am well adjusted socially. YES NO
25. I believe in some kind of Higher Power in my life. YES   NO
26. I think people are basically decent. YES   NO
27. I believe people are evil. YES   NO
28. I think the laws are fair. YES   NO
29. I think the laws are enforced fairly. YES   NO
30. I think I have been treated fairly in my lifetime. YES   NO

Give yourself 1 point for a yes and 2 for a no answer Add the numbers for your total score.
_____
Your score indicates how great an impact your PTSD has had in your lifetime. If your score is between:
5 and 10 the effect is slight.

11 and 20 the effect is somewhat powerful.
Over 20 the effect is powerful.

This will show you how much affect PTSD has on you and how it can disturb you and your relations with others each day. The test is subjective, not scientifically based It merely reflects your relationship with the world.

People who live with PTSD may want and do accumulate many personal possessions. The feeling of loss of control, and helplessness experienced during the trauma, is minimized when possessions are about. They create a feeling of control and permanence. One client, whose wife was a war orphan, discovered when they moved from their home of ten years, caches of food she had put away.

The loss of control and feelings of helplessness experienced by those who have lived through a trauma can create a preoccupation with position. This relates to the need to be somebody, either for the first time, or to reinstate his or her pre-trauma position. The feeling of loss of ability comes from the intense fear trauma brings. The feeling of inadequacy in many areas of your life is a typical reaction if you suffer from PTSD. The response to feeling inadequate creates the Type A personality, the overachiever.

ANGER

Anger is the most consistent and obvious symptom of Post Traumatic Stress Disorder. It shows up in almost everyone suffering from the disorder. Anger ranges from a single simple upset with family, friends and fellow-workers, to old, nurtured hatreds of the government administration, military and civilian leaders. They often express intense fury and at the lack of concern for the environment, and the inadequacies of political leaders. Some are angry about everything. They personalize the unfeeling attitude of healthy drivers who park in handicapped spots, and are unreasonably disturbed by incompetence of uncaring clerks. While the source of their wrath is a reaction to the insult they often become confused at the fury they continue to feel years afterward when they should be enjoying peace and tranquillity.

Once old fears from armed conflict can be connected to disturbing events in civilian life, the uneasiness may be relieved. Combat veterans conditioned themselves to bury thoughts of fear while in a war zone. This habit of making an admission of terror while under fire stays with them. The buried fears, mixed with feelings of concern about possible cowardice under fire, are hard to identify. Sometimes they are so well modified, it is difficult to determine the reality. To create a coping mechanism for such clients becomes extremely difficult.

Indefinable, faded, or out of focus flashbacks create difficult situations to uncover when anger continues to surface without explanation. Many clients speak of "out of body" experiences. Some psychology practitioners share the opinion that a lot of time in combat was spent in this very real state of sub-conscious functioning. Thus the trauma is relegated to a lower level of memory in the sub-conscious. While the reaction is obvious, making the connection is extremely difficult.

Alcohol and drug abuses are frequently the only defense against intrusive thoughts and memories. Those who have suffered trauma may not be able to make the connection between it and chemical abuse.

Ruminating over the cause for his addiction merely creates more puzzlement and frustration. Until a sufferer reaches a willingness to accept the lack of control over drinking or drug use and recovery begins, only then can the therapist and client make headway to uncover the root cause of the anger.

Some make an unrealistic leap from Maslow's defined state of "survival" to "self actualization." Abraham Maslow, a psychiatrist, developed a hierarchy of needs. On the lowest level was survival and safety, basic human needs for life. On the very top level he placed self actualization, a condition in which the person is only interested in helping others. While not an honest motive, some with PTSD continue to express a desire to help others, to correct many social wrongs, cure environmental problems, and offer simplistic suggestions to government and military establishments to fix the wrongs of society. By directing anger at these "great wrongs," emphasis on self dissipates. No longer must the client look in the mirror at his or her own shortcomings. They can speak with fervor about the unknown "they" who cause the difficulties in the world. When all else fails, this anger is directed at large institutions. It stays alive fed by stories of treatment that did not measure up to the impossibly high standards often established by those who demand little of themselves.

Direct confrontation with this unrealistic thinking has proved to be the best way to modify anger from such sources. One client told us he looked hard at himself in the mirror each morning in order to get himself into "The right size to face the world." That action made him realize he did not have to carry the problems of the world on his shoulders.

SEX

PTSD can create major sex problems from unwillingness or inability to become involved in an intimate relationship to continuing lustful pursuits. Lack of interest in sexual intimacy is often the result of unwillingness to get close to another person. PTSD creates a mind set of suspicion and worry about being hurt. This can be as devastating as a loved one leaving the relationship, or as hurtful as the rejection of a simple loving gesture. The capacity to feel tenderness toward another has been destroyed. The anxiety remaining from the time of trauma also contributes to this lack of loving capacity.

This is most obvious in war veterans who connect their sexual experiences in a combat zone with their lives many years later. Among the most obvious and sensitive area is in sexual experience that may have started with prostitutes. They are connected with feelings that involved only immediate gratification. This early exposure and experience sticks with the person when he becomes involved someone who he loves an entirely different manner. Unfortunately, the experience leaves a deep impression that will not allow the husband to approach his wife in as tender and loving manner he would choose. This can lead to many difficult interpersonal situations outside of the wedding bed and beyond the immediate sexual relationships of a man and wife.

INTRUSIVE MEMORIES

Clients have told us about the pain that intrusive memories give them. When they least expect it, just as in a flashback, the memory of the trauma returns. We have all seen those who are discussing a traumatic time with another on television or in person, break down in tears when they talk about them. Even many years later a person will break down while talking casually about a time of great stress in their past. There is a difference between intrusive memories and a flashback. The first is a reaction to overpowering emotion, and the other is an unwelcome recall of a moment in their traumatic past.

MULTIPLE PERSONALITY DISORDER AND PTSD

There are some factors in our work with those who live with PTSD that have raised questions for the researchers to investigate further. One of those is Multiple Personality Disorder. Any number of individual personalities living in one person evidences that disorder. There are some famous cases, including the movies, "Three Faces of Eve", and "Sybil."

From the empirical evidence we have seen in many cases of PTSD, we think there is a definite connection between it and MPSD. The effects of trauma seem to fix a time in the person's life. For instance we know that to a people have been affected deeply by them in traumatic incidents.

Lack of personal discipline can contribute to the perpetuation and intensity of PTSD. That creates the inability to look down the road to a better future. Many have been so traumatized they get stuck in the time of the grim experience. There is a theory that multiple traumas occurring at different times, create multiple personalities and the resulting disorder those many personalities in one person can create.

Because these personality characteristics only show up occasionally, the professional counselor often ignores the dichotomy when current behavior is not age appropriate. The problem is aggravating to partners or associates. It is the task of the therapist to bring attention to this distortion in interpersonal relations, and help change their mental attitudes.

PSYCHIC NUMBING

Psychic numbing or blunting often results from trauma. Trauma victims often describe the aforementioned feeling of detachment from others, and an inability to feel pleasant emotions. This blunting of feeling is well described by
Fritz Wentzel, a commander in the German Navy held prisoner in England during the Second World War who wrote:
> I once saw a ship carrying home men who had been prisoners in the First World War. The sight of those thin haggard-looking men, and the sadness with which they looked down silently at us children gazing up at them in awe has never left me. Now I am as one of them." (1954). [11]

The inability of men to react favorably to admiring gaze of children as they returned to their homeland, shows how much their feelings had been suppressed. Frankl also wrote of this numbing when he described men recently liberated as "not yet liberated in their minds." [5]

This emotional numbing carries on into all interpersonal relationships. On the job, fellow workers are puzzled by the "stand-offish" attitude of one who lives with PTSD. They cannot understand why he or she seems to be lost in another world. While the person may perform his or her duties well, they do not join into the "team" concept." Often, this is shrugged off by, "Well that's just the way she is." Fellow workers tolerate this loner attitude, and by others in social situations, who are unaware that the source of the disposition is a deep-seated mistrust of people, cause in part by feelings of betrayal about the traumatic event.

The attitude is more damaging in a marriage. The warm loving spouse may become a stranger as the result of PTSD. The young wife, who sent her new husband overseas to a war zone, is confused and hurt by the stranger who came back to her. During the Viet Nam war, men were given leave to Hawaii to meet with their wives. These men were taken out of the fighting, cleaned up, and flown to an R and R location in the Islands. Neither they or their wives had any counseling, or time to move slowly back into their relationship. For a short time, their joy at meeting, and their passions carried them along. But in a short time, the stress of battle came between them. The tenderness of their love was invaded by the undiscovered survival patterns that were now part and parcel of their husband's personality. One wife told us she could tolerate being thrown to the floor when he heard a loud noise. But she was totally in the dark as to why he seemed to be on guard all of the time, why he appeared to look for danger everywhere, and carried around a poorly disguised anger at everyone and everything. The personality characteristics that showed up in these short visits of ten days or two weeks were often forgotten.

The complexity and depth of the unpleasant attitudes became unbearable when the men returned to civilian life. As young people can do, they adjusted to the less obvious changes. As long as alcohol, drug or other kinds of interpersonal abuse were not present, the less obvious and more tolerable underlying personality characteristics were tolerated. These traits usually came to the fore when all of the other life problems seemed to be solved. Men were established in their occupations, children were grown and gone from the home, and finances were under control. Now, it seemed life should be good. Unfortunately, it often was not the case. The release of demands for survival of self and the family opened the floodgates of feeling from the old trauma. Those who could not face this disturbing problem fled the situation, not realizing they would take the disorder with them. Some buried it in alcohol or drug abuse. Others left their families, jobs, and friends in a futile attempt to find peace of mind in a new location.

After hitting the bottom of their emotional lives, many were able to recover with the help of professional therapists. Others became the homeless, the drifter, and the lost. All because of a trauma buried in their personal history.

ARRESTED DEVELOPMENT

Intense trauma can cause an arrest of development. The emotional reactions to a situation, perceived as similar to the original trauma, is the same as those experienced during the original trauma. Thus a middle aged person will react as a teenager, or even as a young child. This arrested development can arise in other actions of the victim. His or her interpersonal relations are often out of phase for their calendar age and presumed state of maturity. We have theorized, but have no scientific base for our concept, that trauma causes multiple personalities to exist in the same person. That is to say that one who has suffered a trauma, stops development in that part of their psyche, and reacts as one at that age when a stimulus causes the trauma to come to the conscious mind. Because the victim does not react to all life situations in an inappropriate manner, chaos results, particularly with those closest to the sufferer.

We found this situation with men whose early sexual experiences were with prostitutes. They may have all sort of loving manners toward their wives, be considerate in many ways, and be a model citizen and spouse. But in the bed chamber, the trauma (and that is the right term in these situations) of an early, relatively unsatisfactory and unfeeling sexual experience gets in the way of a reasonably developed sexuality. We are told that the pornographic web sites have more activity, than all of the other retail sites combined. Certainly this would indicate there is a great void in the understanding of reasonable sexuality. The attitude of this section of the public would appear to be one a voyeur rather than a caring and unselfish participant and partner.

CHAPTER THREE

CAUSES

Post Traumatic Stress Disorder is one of those illnesses that insists you do not have it. In part this is because many think those who have a mental disorder are "crazy" (what ever that means). The disorder part, the conscious disturbances that result from PTSD do not show up for months, or even years after the traumatic event that causes it. So, the mental disturbance occurring today is often not connected with the trauma of a yesterday that can be many years back in your personal history.

One's life can be rattling along in good order, except for the usual intermittent problems. One who has lived through a trauma can, on a clear summer day, surrounded by a happy and healthy family, have a flashback of the trauma powerful enough to shatter the pleasant and joyous mood for a day or for a week.

Men who have seen innocent children destroyed in war, find it hard to enjoy watching children play. The impact of seeing dead children returns when they see the joy and laughter of children having fun. The connection in their subconscious is too strong to break, i.e. children at play will be killed and their joy of living will certainly is cut short. So those who live with this thought process will avoid children at play, and may be visibly upset at the merriment without really knowing why.

Concentration camp survivors admit the feeling of responsibility for children is sometimes more than they can handle. They watched as children were separated from their parents in the camps. They felt the hopelessness of the situation and helplessness of parents to protect their child.

As time goes on, the sufferer consciously avoids enjoying the pleasures of life. The fear that such enjoyable times will always be destroyed by the ever present upsetting subconscious memories dulls the ability to take pleasure in life itself.

PTSD is an "out of phase" disorder. Those who suffer with this disorder are people who can no longer identify with their peers. The sense of values they have lived with for years no longer serves them. They complain of feeling "ill at ease," because what has worked for them in the past has lost its validity. Friends, family and co-workers sense the changes, but have no idea how to handle them. The lack of physical complaints confuses everyone. Frustrated at the inability to handle the effects of PTSD causes the patient often rail at the big problems of society. It is much easier to voice concern at the excesses of government, than it is to face the new set of fears that cause loss of sleep, loss of libido, feelings of being all alone, separate and different from peers.

Patients often ask how they have been able to function for many years, without the intense impact Post Traumatic Stress brings to them in their mid life. The explanation is a simple one. As we grow and develop, the social compact expected by society takes over without conscious effort. Psychiatry labels this process "imprinting." Our parents, teachers, and elders tell us how we are expected to act as our life progresses, even to the time of our dotage. We accept this imprinting by osmosis, with little conscious effort. We are expected to get educated, marry, have children, start on a career path, and take on other obligations pressed on us by families, employers, the church and our community. By taking up this charge we consciously and unconsciously put the troubles of the past behind us. The requirements of our day to day life leave little time for us to stare at the past. The effects of trauma, while no longer in our consciousness are nonetheless a part of our thinking. PTSD forces us into actions we do not understand. This unconscious process is not an excuse for anti-social behavior, but it is a major reason for some aberrant behavior. Therapy to relieve the pressures can bring understanding, and hope for relief. We can change when we can uncover, accept and attempt to modify these unconscious but powerful drives.

Once we have suffered a trauma, PTSD continues to hide itself in our psyche. It seems to come to the fore as men and women approach what is loosely termed "middle age." At this time the demands of career, parenthood, and earlier efforts of getting established in a life have passed. This is a time for the relaxation of tensions. One now feels settled, safe and comfortable. A kind of letting down from the stresses of living comes into play. As vitality decreases, physical and psychological burdens can no longer be denied. Memories may return with reinforced strength. The symptoms of PTSD can now force their way into this peaceful scene.

Because those who meet with trauma try to forget the incidents, mis-diagnoses continue to plague suffers of PTSD. Mental health practitioners with no understanding of the results of PTSD, pick out symptoms of mental disturbance with which they are familiar. The usual prognosis is schizophrenia. Many of the difficulties of the schizophrenic are common to one who lives with PTSD. The symptoms of narcissism, paranoia, avoidance, and selective amnesia are part of schizophrenia and of PTSD. The psychologist or doctor often fails to tie these many specifics to the complexity of Post Traumatic Stress disorder.

Difficulties arrive long after the event has faded from conscious memory. The effects, buried in the subconscious, continue to plague those injured. They show up as disturbed sleep; short temperedness; hyper alertness; avoidance of anything that could refresh memories of the trauma; a feeling that life is useless; an unwillingness to make long term commitments; often drug or alcohol abuse; nightmares; and in severe cases, poor judgment, impaired concentration and thought process.

PTSD causes distorted thinking in the sufferers. This result has nothing to do with intelligence, nor does it mean a mental decline. It is simply a distortion in the immediate way one reacts to certain events or people in your life. PTSD, if not diagnosed early after the trauma occurred, may not show up in its most virulent forms for years. During that time the victim can experience many strange or unreasonable reactions to ordinary life events.

Fortunately the symptoms of PTSD can be modified by therapy to understand what happened, and its effect on what is happening now. Experiencing a trauma, and suffering from the results of that trauma, causes those who have lived through it to react in certain ways. Only an experienced therapist can uncover the hundreds of ramifications of Post Traumatic Stress Disorder. Some of these are described in the following paragraphs. If you have PTSD, you will recognize yourself in some of them.

If persons, or groups of persons, cause you to become emotionally disturbed and physically agitated, you may be reacting to an event or series of events in your past that your conscious mind no longer recalls. This creates the "I don't know why, but I just don't like foreigners," or other broadly defined groups. It can be the basis for bigotry or other intolerant attitudes.

PTSD may cause a mental upset when you are in certain geographical locations, experience unusual weather, or find yourself in some types of buildings that are large and overwhelming in their sheer volume of space, or in confined quarters. These conditions can stir memories buried in your subconscious. You may be disturbed by odors, noises, textures, perceived sights, or tastes. These attacks on your senses will be way out of proportion the actual conditions.

Some situations or events over which you have no control cause you great mental distress. You might find yourself greatly upset because no one in authority seems to care about the proper manner to dispose of atomic waste or take proper care of the environment.

You may have trouble sleeping. Your mind continues to ruminate over poorly defined social problems, or constantly ponder personal matters that cannot be immediately resolved. As a result, you find yourself awake almost all night. You may be afraid to go to sleep for the nightmares that can come.

Nightmares of the trauma return nightly or at least on a regular basis. You could cry out, talk in your sleep or physically attack your spouse in the sleep state. Often you will awaken in a sweat. You might have flashbacks, a powerful feeling the trauma is happening again. You experience the feeling of helplessness experienced at the time of the trauma. The terror is with you *right now; it is not a memory.* These feelings often occur during the half sleep when we are in that state of limbo when we are no longer asleep, but yet not fully awake.

The feeling might persist that others are out to get you. This can show up by constant concern that you are being cheated, or that you are not being treated fairly. You might now own a gun or guns, and other weapons. You are in a constant state of alert against what you do not know, but IT is, or THEY are out there and are trying to get you.

You refuse to watch television, go to movies, look at pictures, or read about certain places in which the trauma took place. Again, the conscious memory can be buried so deeply, you cannot determine your anathema to these activities. If the subject should come up in conversation, you generally refuse to talk about it, or become greatly disturbed if you do become involved in a discussion.

You may not be able to remember major parts of the trauma. One who has been caught in a forest fire may not be able to recall the sound of forest fire, the time of day, or how they found themselves in the forest. Someone who survived an earthquake might only remember the noise and dust. Combat veterans speak of the dream like quality of battle, and often can not recall specific events.

Your ability to pursue your job and take care of your person or your surroundings may be markedly diminished. You experience a major reduction in caring about the necessary maintenance of your own life.

You can lose interest in inter-personal relations. This will be evidenced by withdrawal from other people, ranging from merely wanting to be alone much of the time, to totally withdrawing from society. These symptoms can be exacerbated by use of drugs or alcohol. At best, you will feel a detachment from others with whom you have been close.

Long range plans are continually put on hold. Those with PTSD find themselves unable to commit to any demanding future commitments. They simply drift from one day to the next. There is a feeling of a foreshortened future.

You could be constantly angry. Sometimes you feel low grade dissatisfaction with everything and everybody. Often there is real hostility toward the world in general. You seethe inwardly at events and toward people with whom you come in contact, no matter how casual.

You may startle easily. While concentrating on a task or book you may react in an extreme manner, even violently if someone comes up behind you, taps your shoulder, or calls out your name. Because of this hyper-alertness many with PTSD keep arms easily available. One client told us that he is never more than an arm length away from a firearm in his house or car. Others have installed professional or homemade alarm systems to give them warning of approaching danger.

There is often solace in dissociation. In this way, you mentally leave your physical location and relieve the immediate stressful situation for a less demanding mental place. This human trait allows us to avoid pain, either physical or mental by dissociating our body from reality. We are unaware of the fact that our mind has gone to a less stressful place than our body occupies. This is selective amnesia when our mind chooses to forget unpleasantness. Unfortunately, our subconscious absorbs all of the torment our being is suffering.

Meditation, a form of dissociation is not this psychic displacement, but rather a conscious, deliberately calming exercise to find mental peace.

Post Traumatic Stress Disorder is usually the result of being personally involved in an event that involves actual or threatened death or serious injury. It can also be the result of learning about unexpected or violent death, serious harm, or threat of death or injury experienced by a family member or other close associate.

Other causes of PTSD include loss of home by fire or earthquake; the results of military combat, either as a soldier, a combat medic or becoming a prisoner of war; witnessing the violent death or injury of a family member; being involved in a serious automobile accident; living through a violent natural disaster such as a tornado or hurricane; being caught in a riot, surviving an airplane crash, a ship or train wreck; being abused as a child; or being the victim of a violent crime such as rape.

PTSD often appears in those who work in emergency rooms, or the trauma units of hospitals. It is also experienced by professional athletes when they can no longer perform as they once did.

All of these happenings, whether the victim is involved willingly or by mischance, create the conditions for PTSD to arise long after the event. Common to all of these incidents is the suddenness and intensity with which they happen. We know of no training, or conditioning that can avert the reaction to these unexpected events. Even highly trained soldiers tell us the death or dismemberment of a comrade, while expected in combat, often results in PTSD long after the time of the action event. A major injury that ends an athletic career has the same result.

Many who suffer a trauma, get through both the trauma and its immediate aftermath with great courage and seeming serenity. We have all heard friends say admiringly about one who suffered a great loss, "She was so strong during the whole difficult time." Such respect for strength in the face of adversity arises from the American heritage of independence and courage. We create a conscious desire to handle difficulty with a calm composure. That ability to maintain mental equilibrium is a valuable trait.

Unfortunately, the damage to our psyche is not as easily overcome. One associate of ours compares PTSD to an apparent healed over wound that was not cleansed properly. The epidermis seems whole, but beneath the seemingly healthy skin is a festering sore. When a new, even moderate damage happens to that unhealthy part of the body, the bleeding and pain can begin again. We define trauma as an emotional wound. It is a shock or blow causing fright those results in damage to psychological development. In medicine, trauma is defined as a serious injury or shock to the body from violence or an accident. The two definitions are interlocked. Many psychological traumas result from physical damage. The confusion comes when the physical problems have been resolved and you are healed, but the mental anguish continues. Those who suffer from Post Traumatic Stress Disorder, complain about a multitude of symptoms that may seem to have no connection to the physical damage they have endured. They live with problems such as poor sleep patterns, difficulty concentrating, unresolved anger, and feelings of being victimized. These problems show up long after the event that caused them. Because of the length of time that passed, mental health practitioners and physical health care givers often did not connect the symptoms with the problem. Time from the date of the trauma could cover years.

ANNIVERSARY DATES

The anniversary date of a trauma cause deep psychic difficulties. The conscious memory can deal with it by dismissing the problem as "history." The unconscious effect is another story. Beginning sometime before the actual date, you may find yourself ill at ease, short with friends and family, having difficulty sleeping, and drinking or smoking more. You might make efforts to make up for feelings of inadequacy by making unnecessary purchases or taking a trip. These are efforts of the subconscious to compensate for the knowledge of the impending tragedy. Remember your subconscious has no capacity to deal with time or place. The subconscious feels the trauma will be repeated. Your feeling of impending doom is not imagination as far as the psyche is concerned. It is preparing to fight off the trauma that it feels will happen again. Don't look around to find some comfort in your outer world. Realize instead that your unconscious is working overtime. You need to consciously think about what really happened, and count your blessings that you are a survivor. You are no longer a victim of a trauma as you were when it happened. You are not helpless now.

One surprising characteristic of PTSD is the commonality of symptoms, regardless of the event that causes the disorder. It is much like having a broken arm or leg. Whatever caused the fracture is of no consequence. The discomfort is the same whether caused by falling out of a tree, or off a bicycle. The healing cycle depends on the skill of the doctors, and the ability of the physical body to replace bone and tissue.

The development of PTSD follows this pattern. The demands of daily living allow our conscious mind to forget the intensity of the event. We believe that we have put the pain behind us, and to a degree that is true. But, the damage to our unconscious is not healed as easily. We have to attend to the underlying problem. Until the distress of the trauma is faced squarely and realistically, so the tragedy can be consciously dealt with, the problem remains waiting to surface again with its accompanying backlash.

SHIPWRECKS

The ferry, Wahini plied the Waterloo harbor in New Zealand, a short four mile trip. During a particularly strong hurricane, it ran aground, and tipped over. It did not sink, as it struck an underwater reef less than a mile from the landing. Because of the more than forty-five degree tilt of the ferry, it was impossible to launch any life boats. The passengers, feeling safe in their life jackets, jumped into the raging sea and attempted to get to the land which was close by. The surge of the sea prevented them from reaching the beach, so they turned around in an attempt to reach the other shore, about three miles away.

The seas were rough, and the water was cold. Rescuers had to drive about an hour to get to the beach where the survivors would be able to land. When they arrived, guards refused to allow them to approach the beach with their vehicles because they felt the risk was too great. One survivor managed to get up the steep cliffs to the rescuers. When he told them about injured passengers on the beach who had been stripped of their clothing by the sea, freezing, in shock, and injured by the sharp rocks the guards relented.

Many died of exposure. Most of those who came through the disaster refused to ever go on the ferry again. The hulk of the Wahini remained in the harbor as a corpselike reminder of the tragedy, reinforcing the unconscious fears of those who had survived.

THE YARMOUTH CASTLE

In the middle 1970's the Yarmouth Castle, a cruise ship, burned at sea. The ship did not meet present day fire standards, and as a result, the fire, which started amidships, and three decks down, spread rapidly through all of the upper decks. The crew was unable to fight the fire effectively because of the intense smoke generated by burning wood and other materials. Within two or three hours, the entire ship was engulfed in a raging fire.

Eighty seven passengers died either in the fire, or as the result of injuries while jumping from the ship. Fortunately, the Bermuda Star, another cruise ship, came alongside, and launched its lifeboats to rescue the passengers. As the passengers descended ropes and ladders to the rescuing lifeboats, they saw people trapped in burning staterooms, and others die when they struck debris as they jumped.

Survivors flash back to the tragedy. Many refused to go out on the water for years. One woman is haunted by memories of a person, trapped in a stateroom below decks, who could not get the porthole open. This woman has awakened as she begins to break her bedroom window in a dream state attempt to rescue the doomed passenger.

The daughter of a survivor tells of her mother awakening many times in the night to check on her children. She lives with the terror that they are in danger, and she must rescue them. One man has flashbacks of being on deck, smelling the acrid smoke and the unbearable heat of the fire. Another lives with claustrophobia as the result of the fire and the sinking. When he reached the Bermuda Star, a man offered him his stateroom to rest. He could not stay in the confined quarters, fleeing instead to the open deck. His claustrophobia as the result of the shipwreck continues to disturb him.

Just before the ship sunk, as it was totally ravaged by the fire, the burning hulk began to make a sound like a baby crying. Now when a survivor hears that sound it creates flashbacks to the harrowing experience of fire at sea. Mental confusion reigns as the cry of a helpless infant brings back feelings of raw terror. The sound should not normally create alarm. Others are brought back to that frightening night when they smell smoke, even if they know consciously that it is a friendly fire.

On shipboard, one is at the mercy and in the care of the captain and crew. Control is totally in their hands. Shortly after the fire started, the captain and some of the crew abandoned ship. Survivors say that no senior officers remained to take care of the passengers. This abdication of responsibility by the senior authority figure on the ship will recur in later life of the survivors. They may not understand why they do not trust those in command of their fate. It can be as simple a situation as riding a bus, or being in an automobile that someone else is driving. The combination of loss of control, and the feeling of imminent abandonment by the one in control can cause great distress, and deep feelings of anger.

A GERMAN ARMY HOSPITAL SHIP

During World War II a German hospital ship carrying more than 4,000 badly wounded German soldiers from the Russian front, was torpedoed by a Russian submarine in the in the Baltic Sea. Controversy continues about the prominence and lighting of Red Cross markings on the ship, which under International Law would preclude any attack on it.

The surgeons were operating on the wounded when the torpedo struck. The other men were helpless because of their wounds. There was no where near enough medical staff to help more than a few of them to safety. One male survivor, a corpsman, tells of his continuing dreams of the screams of the men as they lay in their beds, knowing they were about to drown. Another survivor, a nurse, cannot even speak about the tragedy without breaking down. The events of that night remain a vivid and unwanted memory, causing her great anguish. She continues to live with feelings of inadequacy and fear of the sea and the dark. She has little confidence in others who are charged with her personal safety.

A NORWEGIAN FERRY SINKING

Norway has hundreds of miles of coastline. Boats and ships are the main method of transportation to and from the villages on the coastline, and across the North Sea. About ten years ago, a new ferry was put into service with a crew of 55 men and women, all well experienced in seamanship. They had worked together for a number of years on other ferries.

On its first voyage, the new ship turned turtle and sank very quickly during a raging storm. The experienced crew was handling a ship that was still strange to them. The inability of the seasoned crew to save the passengers created PTSD in all of them. Therapists worked with them to moderate their distress at failing to perform their rescue duties in what they deemed a proper fashion. They were trained to keep passengers from harm. Their failure to perform that duty continued to disturb them so that some refused to go to sea again. Others continued to be haunted by nightmares about the sinking and the dead passengers.

THE BRITTANIC

A World War I female nurse survived the sinking of the Titanic when she was a young girl. She also survived the sinking of the Brittanic, the sister ship of the Titanic when it was serving the British Navy as a hospital ship. The reason for the sinking of the Brittanic remains a mystery. This survivor suffers a continuing nightmare of her being in her bed while water rushes into her cabin through an open porthole. She is unable to get out of bed to save herself. She awakens shaking and perspiring.

FLASHBACKS

A retired Navy nurse whose military service experience was mainly in orthopedic surgery believed she had put the painful memories of young men's amputated limbs behind her. She suffered an unsettling experience long after her service days. She was a passenger in a car when it passed a number of the white passenger buses used by the Navy and Marine Corps to transport personnel. She became totally overwhelmed by the sight, broke into tears, and cried out to her companion, "No more buses!" The deep seated memory of the buses bringing badly wounded men to undergo surgery that involved amputation, returned causing her great distress The fact that it was a peaceful day, and that the buses had no wounded in them, made no difference to her unconscious. With no warning the anguish of dealing with the suffering of wounded men returned with all of its original intensity.

Research has shown survivors of concentration camps avoid any kind of institutional care because they fear the loss of identity, such as they experienced in the camps.

A former prisoner of war in Germany in his words, "almost went into shock" when a contingent of German officers, who were guests of the sponsoring organization, walked into a banquet he was attending about five years after the end of the war. His reaction was one of total panic. The innocent moment was simply that, but the memory of the experience stayed with him for years.

A senior psychiatrist in a leading hospital, formerly a prisoner of war in Japan, admitted that he had an almost overpowering urge to run his car into any Japanese automobile he met on the street. Again, a momentary, unreasonable reaction, but extremely intense. The experiences left him shaking and in a sweat.

Another case involved a former combat soldier who survived his wounds suffered in a series of terrible battles during the Italian winter. His home is in a wooded area in an area that gets heavy winter snows. The terror, pain of wounds, and fears of inadequacy always come back to him when he looks out of his windows on a cloudy gray day. He told us "I expect the gray coats to move out of the woods at any minute." Of course, his reason takes over, but the power of the situation contributes to his anxiety.

In these instances the person will experience intense mental distress. The body will react and experience the same physical sensations as during the original trauma. This always happens when someone living with PTSD goes through an experience that triggers the long buried memories.

LONELINESS AND WITHDRAWAL

Those who now suffer from Post Traumatic Stress Disorder experienced a trauma for which they were totally unprepared. One encounters a traumatic experience with an ingenuous attitude powerful enough to cause Post Traumatic Stress Disorder. In cases of PTSD particularly in the case of civilian soldiers, the trauma of combat is intensified by at least a relative innocence of spirit. This loss of innocence is easy enough to understand when we become aware of the long term effect of trauma.

PTSD sufferers live with a feeling of being greatly damaged, and that they were totally innocent of any wrongdoing. In this ingenuousness, they adjust in many ways in an unconscious effort to recapture that former purity of heart. The Stockholm syndrome is a perfect example of adjustment, and a self preservation attitude.

Some force themselves to return to the scene. Others do academic research to determine the conditions in which they found themselves and the reasons for the situation. These efforts assist in placing the trauma in a realistic frame. Therapists speak of reframing the experience. The effort is intended to put the trauma in another light in order to see it not in the fog of twisted memory. An insurance company advertisement showed only the outline of a windshield with only white space inside of it. The caption said "Picture of an accident about to happen." A simplistic but accurate portrayal of the difficulty in remembering the details of a trauma. It is vital to become somewhat comfortable with the memories of a trauma to make it real, and make the memory accurate in order to deal with what really happened. Reframing is a technique that attempts to look at the trauma from a different perspective, with an understanding of how distorted the memory can be. It also brings the unconscious fears into the light of reason. This process is very difficult when the client is in denial of the effects of the traumatic incident on their current life. When one thinks of the terms used to describe trauma, the normal inability to create an accurate memory becomes more clear. People who have been traumatized use terms like knocked down, bowled over, flattened, smacked in the face, ambushed, and beaten down.

After the trauma is over, most people try to get on with their life by attempting to put the experience behind them. This conscious effort works for a while. But the unconscious and powerful feeling of betrayal by higher authority, government, the church, and family and even God intensifies the desire to forget the experience. The conscious effort is of little avail. The memory does fade from conscious memory; but the subconscious betrays the conscious by nurturing the effects of the trauma.

FEELINGS OF GUILT, FAILURE, AND INADEQUACY

Among men who fought in Viet Nam, and former prisoners of war from all wars, feelings of failure were constantly expressed. Both groups felt they should have done more, even to the point of being killed in battle. We were unable to determine the deeper source for those feelings, even with the most cooperative of subjects. Men who had been forced to bail out of burning aircraft carried feelings that they were somehow personally responsible for not being able to complete their mission. While they were well aware that their feelings of guilt were irrational, it was impossible to shake the thought that they had failed in some way. The best we could do with such cases was to develop an acceptance that their feelings of guilt were in fact illogical and so should be consciously discarded. In this way, the intensity of their reaction was minimized. It could not be totally erased.

One high ranking officer refused to wear the Prisoner of War Medal because of shame he felt by being captured by the enemy. This was in spite of his years of exemplary service long after his capture and release. Another, who had been brutally treated by his captors, would not apply for any medical help or compensation from the VA. We helped a Viet Nam veteran write his experiences in order to apply for compensation. Once it was completed, he turned himself in to the psychiatric ward in order to recover from the trauma of reliving his personal account of a year in combat. In spite of his honorable service in a combat zone, he believed (and still does) that he had not done enough, or sacrificed what to him was an acceptable amount for his country. He felt shame for not being subjected to danger every day while in the combat zone.

WAR VETERANS

While PTSD was first found in war veterans, it is not limited to those who fought in military actions. Other experiences can cause Post Traumatic Stress Disorder, including being in an automobile accidents; living through an earthquake or a serious fire; surviving an airplane or train crash; living through a shipwreck; being caught up in a riot, or out of control crowd situation. Being raped or attacked by animals; finding yourself the target of an indiscriminate shooting; working as a paramedic, serving as a nurse or doctor in an emergency room; discovering a victim of suicide; and living through armed combat are all sources of PTSD. Men and women who were concentration camp inmates and those who were prisoners of war all live with the effects of PTSD.

The common thread in these events is they are all beyond any usual human experience. They often involve lightning quick, and life threatening experiences. Innocents usually endure the events. Even the combat soldier feels a vulnerability and guilt based on childhood teaching of respect for life. Others doing their chosen jobs are impacted by traumas not of their making, whether they are the victim, an observer, or become a caregiver. These innocents bear the damage they suffer, wondering what happened. The psyche tenderly and mysteriously allows them to forget the intensity soon after the event, when they cannot believe these terrible out of the ordinary circumstance happened to them. While this psychological defense mechanism offers relief, the trauma remains deeply implanted in the subconscious. The subsequent effects cannot be related to the trauma. We will discuss some of these reactions in following chapters.

Experiencing or observing a trauma creates a powerful impact on both our conscious and subconscious. The effects of the horror remain long after the happening. Even in the face of trauma, we apparently able to continue functioning. Afterwards we remove the event from our conscious memory in order to help and comfort the injured, others or ourselves. We try to put the occurrence behind us so we can get on with our lives. In our conscious mind we have done so, but the subconscious retains the pain and agony of the event.

CHAPTER 4

COPING WITH PTSD

We would be arrogant indeed if we proposed there were cures for PTSD. Just as the addictive person is never "cured," neither is the person who lives with PTSD. Someone has said "You cannot kill your demons, you can only educate them."

What we have accomplished with these people is to develop an understanding of their disorder. In short, we attempt to find the cause, look at it critically and realistically; then connect that trauma with their actions and reactions to their lives today. This understanding and acceptance allows them to understand that their unusual responses to stimuli are the result of old experiences buried in their unconscious. By developing this insight we relieve the discomfort of the immediate and usually unacceptable reaction with comprehension and modification of their conduct.

We find that the reactions are so deeply ingrained that clients will wonder why they react in such a manner. It is the job of the therapist to help uncover the details of the trauma to clarify the incident. Memory is fallible, and memory of trauma is usually unreliable. The distortion comes from the unwillingness of the conscious mind to accept the horror of the event. On the other hand, the unconscious holds all of its frightening detail. This dichotomy creates the confusion and consternation. The person is aware they suffered a trauma; a natural disaster, an accident, or a wartime experience. They could have been involved personally, or they have seen such an incident. Either way, their minds were impacted and left damaged by the scene and their unconscious records it forever.

Denial is major factor in the unwillingness or inability of someone with PTSD to remember accurately what happened. Denial is both a conscious and unconscious reaction to an occurrence. If a person is living with Post Traumatic Stress Disorder, the denial must be replaced with acceptance to relieve the symptoms.

Once the acceptance is accomplished, we have followed a process of replacing old ways of reacting with new ways of looking at their lives. This hopefully gives them a change in their perception of events in their lives—that they are presently reacting in a manner out of date, obsolete, and unusable in their life today.

Most people living with PTSD tend to isolate, to avoid social contact even to the extent of becoming separated emotionally from their wives and family. Some of this can be from early training and imprinting that happened before the time of trauma. PTSD will accentuate this personality characteristic. Many people are unaware of the need to improve their communication skills.

We have used the following set of helpful techniques to alleviate the isolation. They are particularly effective in groups but can be used by individuals either as part of therapy or by self instruction. Part of the concept is that difficulties with communication are widespread. A person should not be embarrassed because of an inability to communicate effectively. Communicating well can be learned. Do not expect that merely reading this kind of list can solve your communication difficulties. Be aware if how you react presently, and attempt to change the way you handle your interpersonal relationships. There are many blocks to clear effective communication with others. The blocks get in the way of healthy, creative relationships and therefore interfere with intimacy and warmth with others, especially mates, family, friends and associates.

The following guidelines are useful in assisting individuals in becoming more "open" and able to give and receive clear communication with others and potentially avoid confusing and ineffective communication.

1. SPEAK WITH THE FIRST PERSON "I". Instead of "people feel" or "you get to feeling. . ." etc., say, "I think, I feel. . ." such and such. This gives more of the flavor of you rather than broad generalities.

"You" statements are generally perceived as blaming and confrontational. A person tends to shift into a defensive state the moment there is a suggestion of blame being thrust upon them. Defensiveness stops the flow of clear, open communication.

Avoid using absolutes such as "always" and "never". This simply isn't true and it can be perceived as punishing, condescending, controlling, etc.

2. Good communication involves clear expression of not only what you think and feel, but also the ability to listen clearly to the words, feelings and behaviors communicated by another. (It is good to attempt to occasionally "crawl into another's skin" or "wear their moccasins" in your imagination in order to understand the individual.). There is a strong tendency to "read in"

things we feel while missing what the person is really attempting to convey. We also tend to "read out" or ignore things a person is expressing because it bothers us for some reason. Techniques such as repeating back to a person what you thought he said before you answer might be helpful if it does not dampen spontaneity. One can learn to allow for one's biases and prejudices which may distort what is happening in and around us.

Be aware of a tendency to consistently interrupt another person. This often occurs at a critical point in a discussion.

4. SPEAK DIRECTLY TO INDIVIDUALS. Look and speak directly into their face(s). For example, if another person asks you: "How do you feel about Bill right now?" turn to Bill and say, "Bill, I feel you were very kind to me a minute ago when you said. . .", or "I resent you right now" or whatever - rather than answering the one who originally questioned you.

Remember to have good eye contact with the individual with whom you are communicating.

5. SPEAK FROM YOUR HONEST FEELINGS AND THOUGHTS. Failing to communicate exactly what one feels -- (i.e., anger, affection or indifference) -- toward another is deemed "kindness" by the world and all too often is the most cruel thing we can do to another. It is based on lying and not paying a person the compliment of being able to handle honest feelings. How can persons behave properly if they have never honestly been told how others react to them?

Remember: Speaking your truth doesn't automatically license a person to be aggressive, domineering, condescending, rude, mean or just plain nasty in communicating with other people. Effective communication is best achieved when an individual maintains consistent empathic behavior toward others.

6... MAKE AN ACTIVE AND HONEST EFFORT TO BE AWARE OF YOUR THOUGHTS AND FEELINGS IN THE MOMENT. This is difficult initially, however, with practice and lots of patience this can be achieved. The important point is to express your thoughts and feelings at the earliest appropriate time. Be aware even if you cannot express a perception in the moment. We cannot live creatively in the present if we cloud the present with past memories. The dreamed-of future never comes. We freely live in only one dimension of time - the here and now.

Identify your emotions as a <u>signal</u> and not a truth. Emotions often have a prejudicial attachment to an encounter, especially if a person is determined to "win" a point or a disagreement, etc.

7. READ THE MESSAGES FROM YOUR OWN BODY. Your body is a most basic, tangible aspect of yourself. It is continually giving you messages. The opened or closed position of your limbs, sweating palms, feeling "fidgety,'" rapid heartbeat, rapid breathing, moving to a closer or more remote seat, flushed face, increased elimination needs - all these and more may tell you that you are afraid, angry, irritated, worried, embarrassed, wanting to be closer to a person, anxious, etc. These messages can be noted and explored when timely and appropriate.

8. BE AS SPONTANEOUS AS POSSIBLE. Too often people "mull over", think about, choose careful language, wait too long, try to be polite, or censure what they want to say or how they want to honestly react. This may "water down" and negate one's freshness, sparkle and genuineness. Let ideas, thoughts and feelings be expressed as they will convey the true "you."

9. STAY WITH THE ISSUE AT HAND. In communicating with another individual it is easy to digress, get lost in words, etc. and miss the focus of the issue being examined. "Wandering communication" is often a defense/resistance against something that needs to be addressed or expressed.

10. BE AWARE OF THE ROLES YOU TAKE AND YOU'RE CHARACTERISTIC BEHAVIOR. It has been observed that we tend to behave similarly in most instances. For example, some people appear to be prepared to do battle at any time. Others tend to withdraw or run away from a confrontation while others become "peacemakers" or "compromisers". Further, there are people who behave very differently in almost every situation, so that they belong. By observing yourself and others you can come to helpful insights about yourself.

11. BE AWARE OF HOW INDIVIDUALS REMIND YOU OF OTHER SIGNIFICANT PEOPLE IN YOUR PAST OR PRESENT LIFE. For instance, a certain person may remind you of your father/mother, or your wife/husband or an old girlfriend/boyfriend. Interacting with those persons offers an opportunity to work out old problems,

affections, hurts, joys, sorrows, etc. even if the person is not actually or completely like the person of whom you are reminded.

12. DON'T SPEAK FOR OTHERS. Such as: ". . . most men think. . .," "a man always feels. . .," "I think Bill feels you don't like him. . .," etc. Speak for yourself or ask the person what he/she is feeling or thinking. If you feel empathy for a person, or feel like defending or attacking someone, speak for what you are experiencing at that moment rather than projecting or displacing your own feelings off onto others. Further, the use of "we" in most interactions is generally not appropriate.

13. TRY TO HAVE GENUINE "INTERACTIONS" WITH OTHERS. The aim of interaction is not necessarily to fight, to be on good terms, or to "love" everyone. Instead, it is to realize that the basic stuff of life is to contact, interact, feel and communicate meaningfully with others. A quarrel is often better than complacency or ignoring another. To know that you have been true to yourself while meaningfully interacting with another who is being true to himself/herself is a major aim of such an experience as this. It can have favorable consequences in all aspects of your life.

A SIMPLE RULE TO FOLLOW IS TO "SAY WHAT YOU MEAN AND MEAN WHAT YOU SAY".

14. EXPECT PERIODS OF SILENCE. Although silence may seem uncomfortable at first, nevertheless, creative things can occur in our awareness and consciousness. Use silence to be aware of what is

happening in you. In moments of silence take time to "track" your thoughts and feelings.

It is important to not use silence as a "weapon" to win your point or to punish. There are inappropriate uses of silence.

15. BE PREPARED TO ENGAGE YOUR OWN VULNERABILITY. After an emotionally charged discussion or confrontation a variety of feelings, awareness and anxieties are sometimes likely to present. Remember growth occurs via the willingness to be honest and vulnerable.

16 PRACTICE RESPONDING RATHER THAN REACTING. When emotionally charged material surfaces in a discussion it is important to avoid taking a defensive stance. This type of communication takes place at an immature (child) level. It also circumvents personal responsibility. It is <u>reactive communication</u> that impedes mutual, honest, and open interaction. This level of communication predisposes to blaming, ignoring, manipulating, bullying, etc.

The most effective method of communicating is to maintain a mature perspective -- even when the discussions evoke uncomfortable feelings. Deal with the uncomfortable feelings first. This can be done at a mature level. Respond to what is said -- Don't React! Reacting decreases the possibility of being heard. If you feel defensive, talk about that first. Again, <u>you</u> are mutually responsible for creating effective communication. Remember, "RESPONSIBILITY" is merely the "Ability to Respond."

TAKE A GOOD LOOK AT YOURSELF

In a time of personal discovery, we need to ask ourselves questions such as "Who am I?" "What is this all about?" This is the time to look honestly at our past. Remember, the past is prologue. We cannot change the past, only our perception of what happened. Spend the time now:

1. To explore the closets of the mind in which the traumas have been stored. We offer therapy to bring reality to the memory. Our stored memory of trauma always makes it larger, smaller noisier, longer, shorter, and much more terrifying than it has to be now.

2. To begin to make amends to you and to others. Accept the reality of your part in the trauma. We re not speaking of blame, but rather your perception of blame, the one we were taught in our childhood. Look at it realistically, and get on with your life. We must live in reality.

3. To uncover the script of our life we have followed so blindly. As we develop in the phases of our lives, we follow a pattern that was determined in great part by our family and teachers. Do you feel you have betrayed these people by the abrupt change in your life the trauma created? Is the script so pure that it cannot be abandoned if necessary?

4. To create a new set of standards with which to live and measure your life's success. This is a time to doubt, not yourself, but what family and society appear to have expected of us. It is a time to

reappraise what we want from our lives. We cannot live the afternoon of our life by following the program of the morning. Do not bring the rules of the first half our lives into the second half. They no longer apply, and usually do not work.

5. To make a total reality check, to allow the movement from the image of youth to the image of the elder. All major events in our lives whether good or bad, offer us wisdom. Look at the trauma to see what the lessons learned can be. Accept this change as a gift toward more peaceful living.

6. We need to look at our Shadow side, because from the shadow comes the pieces of the puzzle that show us who we really are. Such living is proof of our ability to function in Jung's "tension of the opposites." Jung felt the impetus in our lives came from the shadow side. We need to accept the power in our unconscious for the good it can do for us.

7. We must look past our faults, both real and perceived, to accept ourselves as we really are. We must work to make the changes necessary so we can live the rest of our lives in harmony with others and ourselves. Again, determining and accepting the reality of the trauma is part of this process.

EMOTIONAL STABILITY INVENTORY

Make a self evaluation of your emotional stability by answering these questions, preferably by writing the answers down.

What do I really want out of life?

What do I really expect out of life?

What are the positive attitudes I hold toward life.

What are the negative attitudes I hold toward life.

What have I accomplished in my life?

What do I really want out of life?

What are my present capabilities?

What is my improvement potential?

How do I see myself as a person?

How do I think others think of me?

Which is more realistic?

Which is most important?

MAKE AN HONEST EVALUATION OF:

The mistakes I have made in the past.

Breakdowns in relationships.

Professional or occupational errors.

Failure to meet my own expectations.

Expectations by me that were unrealistic.

Expectations of me by others that were unrealistic.

Examine:

Present financial situation.

Projected financial situation. 1 year-5 years.

Present earning capacity.

Future earning capacity.

Set out in writing:

Long term goals (as long as ten years into future).

Short term goals (as short as one day).

Determine what damage control is needed now:
To correct yesterdays damage.

To forestall future damage.

How much help do I really need?

Where will it come from?

Where have I received help in the past?

Do I have to believe in something outside of me?

What "WHAT IF'S" really tear me up?

Are they real or imagined?

How do I eliminate the "What ifs?"

Where is my ego in all of this?

Do I need all of this ego to survive?

If not for survival, what for?

Do I think of myself as a survivor or a martyr?

How much of myself am I really giving to life?

How much am I truly willing to give to life?

Can I be a self-contained person?

Look at your life from these standpoints:

How important is this (whatever is happening or happened) to me anyway?

Is it life threatening?

Are there any long term physical effects that cannot be repaired?

Is this going to damage me mentally, and if so can it be repaired?

Again, the vital necessity to look at our lives and past events honestly and realistically. One has to get real. Recognize and make a conscious effort to understand what has happened to him/her, and be willing to make the sometimes painful changes necessary to live comfortably.

You can turn the self-centeredness of PTSD to your advantage in working on recovery from trauma. Hillel said, "If I am not for myself, who will be for me? And if I am only for myself, what am I? And if not now--when?" William James said, "Change your life by starting immediately, doing it flamboyantly, with no exceptions." Take the wisdom of these learned men and use it to your advantage, and for the betterment of your life. Only you can make and accept the changes in your attitudes. Others can help, but the final action is yours.

HERE ARE SOME PRINCIPLES TO LIVE BY

➢ Make a commitment to find your true self. Never let anything or anyone stand in the way of that commitment.

➢ Take responsibility for your life. Blame no one. You are the creator of your experience. Your thoughts will manifest themselves in your life in some form. If you do not like the direction your life is taking, change your thinking. Replace negative thoughts with uplifting, positive ones.

➢ Give up giving reasons or excuses. They do not relieve guilt. Self-pity is a waste of time. Accept and forgive yourself and others continuously.

➢ Keep things simple. Always tell the truth. Be polite, it's a kindness to you.

➢ Comparisons have little value. Make no judgments. It is not right or wrong; it just is. Be understanding. Trust that all is that it should be. Remember everyone is coming from the best place they know.

➢ Live in the present. Don't clear away the wreckage of the future.

➢ Spend time alone. Strive for balance and clarity. Appreciate each day.

➢ Do something. There is freedom and peace in action.

➢ In order to live free and happily, you must sacrifice boredom. It is not always an easy sacrifice.

There is no known cure for PTSD. Those who suffer with the effects of this disorder can hope only to find the reasons for their discomfort, to then understand and accept that uneasiness as part of their lives. We ask them to get outside of themselves to see where they fit in the trauma, and to talk with other survivors. We recommend a course of acceptance and a grasp of the reality of the disorder; to deal with what is disturbing today. And very importantly, to learn new reactions to old stimuli.

You will never get rid of the reactions to your trauma. Your unconscious is like a hard drive on a computer. It never forgets the input. The hard drive will keep the information forever. You are not consciously aware of what is in that electronic file. That may seem a cold statement, but it is true. The bright side of the situation is that you can modify the reaction to the old trauma, and thus limit the effect on your daily living.

Use the effects of the trauma itself to build strengths in you. Do not fear your flashbacks. They can be a source of useful information to help you deal with the reality of the trauma you suffered. Explore your nightmares in the cold light of day. They really cannot hurt you in spite of the extreme discomfort they cause.

Let the past lie. Do not dwell on the traumas of yesterday. Look back only to clarify your memory of the trauma in your own mind. By better defining them, you can now deal with them. The reactions caused by buried memories will no longer confuse and anger you.

Here are what some others who have been there have to say about peace of mind:

William Mahedy who was an Army chaplain serving in Viet Nam recommends these steps "For coming out of the night."

1. Shed Hatreds
2. Walk away from violent attachments and violent behaviors.
3. Make a personal moral inventory of those one has harmed.
4. Take action in the face of hatred and anger.
5. Attempt consistent and habitual peace in life (as in your family).
6. Willingly enter the "Cloud of Unknowing" with God.
7. Make a transition from "My God, My God" to "Into your hands".
8. Contemplate just letting life be.
9. Make your prayers forceful and demanding.
10. Become a peacemaker.

This prayer of St. Francis is familiar to us all. Read it with your agonies in mind. His prayer was to help him get outside of his own problems.

> Lord, make us instruments of your peace.
> Where there is hatred, let us sow love;
> Where there is injury, pardon;
> Where there is discord, union;
> Where there is doubt, faith;
> Where there is despair, hope;
> Where there is darkness, light;
> Where there is sadness, joy.

Grant that we may not so much seek
to be consoled as to console;
to be understood as to understand;
to be loved as to love.
For it is giving that we receive;
It is in pardoning that we are pardoned; and it is dying that we are born to eternal life.

THE FEELING OF LOSS AS THE RESULT OF TRAUMA

PTSD is in part the result of a sense of loss. Loss of control, loss of innocence, loss of a sense of invulnerability, and so a loss of peace of mind. This sense is often buried, and not remembered.

Therefore, to ease Post Traumatic Stress, one needs grieving to ease the agony of the disorder. You cannot alleviate the stress alone. A third party is needed but you have to do a lot of the work yourself before you can be helped. The philosopher Rollo May reminds us that "One must face loneliness and anxiety square on. We are all alone."

Jones and Cherry in Grief Recovery Handbook [12] recommend that we gain awareness of the grief we are feeling. Further, if you really are responsible in any way, accept it. Then identify and accept that there is a recovery concept, and you can recover from trauma. And finally, take some action to get your life restarted by moving beyond the loss.

By taking these actions you learn and accept the necessity to replace any guilt caused by the loss of innocence with positive action.

Someone has said about trauma and the guilt we might feel from it, "Claim it/own it/dump it." Start your life over again today.

Kubler-Ross defined the five steps toward recovery from grief. While her work was with the survivors of the death of a loved one, it is our opinion that suffering a trauma is very much like a death experience. Her steps toward recovery from the loss are:

- Denial-we do not want to accept the reality of what happened.
- Anger-we are furious that it happened to us.
- Bargaining-we begin to bargain with ourselves and our God to alleviate the sense of guilt.
- Depression-we fall into a feeling of "what's the use?" and/or life is ended.
- Acceptance-we accept the reality of what happened by reframing the trauma with the help of others if necessary.

After acceptance of the reality of the situation, we can restart our life at peace with ourselves. These are some other thoughts that we offer our clients in order to help them understand the effects of trauma. We do not demean the pain they feel, but others have lived through trauma. These expressions of wisdom are from those who lived through trauma have passed on to us.

We know that to live with PTSD we have to change. Change is not easy or simple. But if one is to find peace of mind, change of attitude is a vital step.

Saul Alinsky who was an early day labor leader as an old man was asked if he thought he had changed.

He said:
    Of course I have changed. There are many who go through the years without

changing. . . (but) life is an adventure of passion, risk, danger, laughter, beauty, love, and a burning curiosity to go with the action to see what it is all about. Most people just exist; they turn from turbulence of change, and try to hide in their private make-believe harbors.

Recovery from the effects of PTSD is a lonely process. It is necessary to contemplate many factors in ourselves, which is often a painful process. But others have done it and you can too.

In the poem Golgotha, Frederick Lawrence Knowles says:

Our crosses are hewn from different trees,
But we all must have our Calvaries;
We may climb the height from a different side,
But we each go up to be crucified;
As we scale the steep, another may share
The dreadful load that our shoulders bear,
But the costliest sorrow is all our own—
For on the summit we bleed alone.

The feeling of loss does not go away in just one attempt. It can seem that just about the time you have reconciled yourself with the effect of trauma, something in your life will change. Be prepared to go back over the landscape of your agonies again if necessary. We do know it is easier the second time. While Father Blake speaks of mid-life, it is our opinion that so called mid-life crises are not a function of age, but rather a function of our moral and spiritual development. Thus they will happen a number of times in our lives.

Sol Alinsky said, "Burn your bridges behind you because you are not going back anyway." In other words live your life to the fullest.

The old curmudgeon George Bernard Shaw wrote:

> This is the true joy in life, the being used for a purpose recognized by yourself as a mighty one; the being a force of nature instead of a feverish selfish clod of ailments and grievances complaining that the world will not devote itself to making me happy.
>
> I want to be thoroughly used up when I die, for the harder I work the more I live. I rejoice in life for its own sake. Life is no brief candle to me. It is a sort of splendid torch which I have got hold of for a moment, and I want to make it burn as brightly as possible before handing it on to future generations.

It is a truism that our mental attitude affects both our mental state as well as our physical being. In American Caesar, General Douglas MacArthur is quoted from one of his speeches to the Corps of Cadets at West Point.

> The years may wrinkle the skin, but to give up interest wrinkles the soul. You are as young as your faith, as old as your doubt; as young as your self confidence, as old as your fear; as young as your hope, as old as your despair. In the central place of every heart there is a recording

chamber; so long as it receives messages of beauty, hope, cheer and courage, so long are you young. When your heart is covered with the snows of pessimism and the ice of cynicism, then and then only are you grown old – and then indeed, as the ballad says, you just fade away. [14]

In our search for peace of mind, we sometimes become too serious in our quest. An unknown author offered this light-hearted recipe for peace of mind.

If I had my life to live over, I'd try to make more mistakes next time. I would relax, I would limber up. I would be sillier than I have been on this trip. I know of very few things that I would take seriously.
I would be crazier, I would be less hygienic.
I would take more chances. I would take more trips.
I would climb more mountains, swim more rivers, and watch more sunsets.
I would eat more ice cream and fewer beans.
I would have more actual troubles and fewer imaginary ones.
You see I am one of those people who live prophylactically and sensibly and sanely,
Hour after hour, day after day.
Oh, I have had my moments and, if I had it to do over again, I'd have more of them.
In fact, I'd have nothing else.

One client told us he had begun to live as well as he could with the problems and limitations of PTSD.

He wrote this to us:

The memories in my mind fade.
The feelings in my heart grow.
And I am at peace with the exchange.

Remember the steps to perfect maturity are immature and imperfect. We can only try, fall down, get up, and try again. The value is in the effort, in the joy of the journey.

Everyone is different as the result of trauma, even those who have come to grips with the changes in their lives afterwards, and made the necessary adjustments to live with the results of those traumas. If one does feel different from others, think on what Henry David Thoreau wrote:

"If a man does not keep pace with his companions, perhaps it is because he hears a different drummer. Let him step to the music which he hears, however measured or far away."

We do not want to wear you out with quotations, but here is a little of Oriental philosophy. The wisdom of the ages is valuable because it has stood the test of time.

The seven emotions and the seven injuries are:Happiness, Anger, Sadness, Fear, Love, Cruelty, and Desire.
Excessive happiness injures the heart
Excessive anger injures the liver
Excessive sadness injures the lungs
Excessive fear injures the gall bladder

Excessive love injures the spirit
Excessive cruelty injures sensitivity
Excessive desires injure the spleen
(Cultivating Stillness, Wong, 1992 p. 42)

We should not sell our ideals short for the sake of expediency or selfishness.... Human law is imperfect. There will always be unprecedented circumstances. Thus we must go beyond rules and operate instead from pure wisdom. We must act with experience, flexibility, and insight. let us so absorb integrity--experience both its triumphs and defeats--that we do the right thing intuitively. Tradition is first. Mercy is greater than tradition. Wisdom is greater than mercy. (Daily meditation, Deng Ming-Dao, 1992)

THE VALUE OF THERAPY

There is a need for curiosity on the part of the sufferer to proceed with therapy. In therapy, a non-victim thought process must be developed. Those who have suffered trauma have a need to grieve—a need to grieve for the loss of innocence, and for those who died in the time of trauma.

We recommend an effort to find a spiritual attitude. This does not mean joining an organized religion, although that may be a way to do it. But rather to look inward to find the power that keeps our lives going.

Again, find the strength that surviving the trauma gave you. In spite of the damage done, there is always a message of strength that comes out of tragedy. Look for it in your meditations, and use that strength.

In the process of understanding what trauma has done to you, and in the process of reorganizing your life it is acceptable to be selfish. Now is the time to take care of yourself and your needs. Ask your spouse or significant other to help you by allowing you time and space to heal. Do not be so self centered that you ignore the needs of others, but that can be taken care of with simple courtesy. Those who live with PTSD must develop the capacity to take care of their own problems before they can take on those of others.

Professional therapists can use hypnosis therapy that helps lower the barriers to memory. They might use behavioral modification combined with cognitive understanding. Those processes use our common sense to understand what is happening to us, combined with new ways of reacting to stimuli. The question of "What causes me to do this?" is a good one to find the underlying reasons for reactions to people, places and things.

BENEFITS AFTER TREATMENT

A stable attitude toward living can bring success to those who felt it would never happen. We have seen men and women, who were lost in this world, find peace of mind, take a new tack in their lives, and achieve success that they never thought could happen, once they were able to understand and cope with their PTSD.

With success came the ability to earn better incomes, live in harmony with their families and fellow workers, and reap the bounty of their new attitudes. We do not hold with the idea that possessions bring happiness, but the lack of financial pressure can make living a lot easier. With financial stability, comes a feeling of inner pride.

We found a high incidence of PTSD in one large group of men who had been prisoners of war. In spite of that, they achieved greater financial returns, had longer marriages, and more stable lives as defined by their attitudes toward their former captors, and society as a whole than those surveyed who had not gone through that kind of traumatic experience. One of the most impressive factors their personality and attitudes reflected, was an acceptance of the affect of their personal problems, yet they had great concern for others, primarily their families. They put the past behind them, recognized they had some old baggage they continued to carry, but found satisfaction in taking their place in society. Their attitudes helped them conduct their own therapy.

A NOTE TO THERAPISTS

Merely to bring old reactions to consciousness is not enough. The patient must be willing to address them, to eventually put them behind him. Another who refused to leave his house on the anniversary of a pitched and bloody battle has cognitively accepted his unrealistic fears and is able to face them. An unreasonable fear of flying was linked to the trauma resulting from an attack by protesters when the client entered the San Francisco airport upon his return from Viet Nam. Some clients, who become irate no matter how gently one probes their actions, may know their actions or reactions are unrealistic. However, they are unable to cope reasonably or to change the behavior. The task of the therapist is to help make the connection, dispel the irrational thoughts and eliminate the old behavior patterns.

Once a patient cognitively accepts the anger source, behavior modification, including repetitive exercises or rituals can help minimize the effect of the stimuli. Most troublesome to modify are actions triggered by unknown stimuli. It becomes necessary to follow the thread of Ariadne, the Greek mythological search, through the jungles of Viet Nam, the deserts of the Persian Gulf, the cities of Somalia, or the sites of civilian trauma. If the therapeutic alliance is strong, the client will assist. A too frightened client will place a greater burden on the therapist to lead the quest. The therapist needs to confront, dig, and with care, force the client to open doors long closed.

Current patterns of behavior offer clues to find the causes for outbursts of rage. Those who have served overseas in combat zones often refer to "The world outside" when speaking of home. This feeling of estrangement recurs when differences arise in domestic situations. Veterans who found distrust, or coldness upon their return from war will close down their emotions again when confronted by what they interpret as abandonment. Sometimes it is necessary to go back to childhood experiences to find the source of the fear of being alone.

In these situations, hypnotherapy and guided imagery is a valuable tool. Unfortunately, the suspicion and apprehension that are part of the disorder can often preclude use of these techniques. Even if the trauma is not fully identified or defined, relief is often the result.

The crux of successful treatment for Post Traumatic Stress disorder for the anger felt by many with PTSD... To find the anger, uncover the fear.

Discovering the denied fear is the most important task of the therapist. Once uncovered, treatment can begin to mitigate this most debilitating expression of buried and often forgotten fear. Then, and only then, can the client expect to reduce the effect of the post trauma stress on his present day life.

WHAT ELSE YOU CAN DO FOR YOURSELF

Find out whom you are really mad at and do something constructive about it. Often when we are disturbed by our spouse, children, fellow workers, we are really being ticked off by events buried in our unconscious.

Our unconscious can cause us difficulty in loving, of being close to another person. It can keep us from caring about other people. When men or women have complained about their love life, we often ask them how they approach their spouse or significant other. The usual answers show they have distorted ideas of how to show affection and love. We have asked men, "When did you last simply touch your loved one's hand? Or when, without any expectation of reciprocal action, did you last say, "I love you." Too often we find the client expects too much from the other person. There is no giving without expectation of a reward of some sort. They cannot find it in themselves to be unselfish. That is the result of trauma, where self preservation and survival were so important. Giving affection and consideration to another person is a great step in restoring and reestablishing them in spite of the shattered assumptions, perceptions of themselves as a victim.

Not only do those who have lived through trauma need to reframe the incident but also there is a need to reframe their concept of themselves in society. This requires self appraisal, and change of attitude. It may require a change in occupation or residence. That process eliminates the old script of whom and what a person thinks he/she is. They can start again with the layer of safety, as defined by Maslow, to build all of the other characteristics of a meaningful life.

Getting outside of oneself is the biggest change needed. One of the characteristics of PTSD is self-centeredness, even to the stage of narcissism. By developing an attitude of concern for others, not only is the concern with self minimized, the process of moving through another phase of moral development occurs. The whole idea is to develop a mature attitude rather than the immature, frozen concept of self that may come with trauma.

These changes also require an acceptance of personal vulnerability. In the twelve step program of Alcoholics Anonymous and other twelve step programs there is a lot of time devoted to accepting humility. Humility is a complex concept, but suffice to say, it involves accepting one's place in society. The need for self esteem is a vital factor in peace of mind. If self esteem is intact, then humility comes easily. One no longer have to put up barriers to protect from the real or imagined "slings and arrows of outrageous fortune."

One technique that has proved itself with war veterans is setting up a group who are willing to go through a debriefing process. Trauma intense enough to cause PTSD, overpowers all other emotions. Group debriefing helps the participants to integrate their lives into an understandable whole. Many therapy groups are out there to help. The idea of these groups is to allow those involved to put their experience into "It was but one period in my life" framework. While the combat experience is extremely stressful and intense, it is not the total of a person's life and should be put in proper perspective. While it was an intense peak it should not be allowed to run his present life in an entirely different place and time. The old patterns of survival in combat no longer apply.

In that kind of group therapy we encourage being gentle with oneself and to eliminate blame as much as possible. We want people to talk about the event in order to reframe, but not to wallow in the event. The idea is to accept the reality of the events, to make them real, to eliminate the distortions of memory. In group work we find this process happens more easily than in one on one sessions. Members find that others have lived with the endorphin rush of sports, or of combat. They begin to realize that others have experienced that mental high, and that they too miss it. They recognize in others the mental and physical exhaustion after the battle, whether sport or armed combat is part of everyone's makeup and memory.

We work toward developing a perception of his or her world as meaningful and comprehensible. We help to find meaning in their new world in order to minimize the distorted memories as much as possible. We try for acceptance of a coherent life. There is great difficulty in understanding overwhelming events like the Holocaust, or the natural disasters of earthquake or volcanic eruption.

In the process we hold out the prospect of worthiness of person, and finding a purpose in the trauma or loss. Then a person can view their life in a positive light.

They can find the ability and strength to restore and reestablish themselves in spite of the shattered assumptions, perceptions. Such shattering that happens when the realization comes that one is no longer capable of continuing in present status. Soldiers are no longer physically or mentally capable of continuing in a combat unit. Athletes no longer can handle the physical demands of their professional position. Professionals find they are unable to handle the demands of their position. Knowing that one's mental or physical capacity is in decline is a terrifying realization. It inflicts a terrible damage to self esteem. That damage needs repairing using therapy to accept the present limitations, and to offer and embrace this new way of life with equanimity and dignity.

CHAPTER FIVE

CASES AND TREATMENTS

The unpleasant effect of any life event is usually stored in the conscious memory. In time all memory fades, and as many say, "it is like a dream." This kind of memory can be brought back to the conscious memory. While details may be lost, the event or situation is recalled with relative ease. Unpleasant memories, embarrassing situations such as failure to perform well in school or at work, are not the debilitating memories stored in the unconscious that cause PTSD. Such distressing memories may cause us to blush inwardly, or to hope no one else remembers the event. But they are like mosquito bites compared to a broken leg when compared to the incidents that create the elements that end up as Post Traumatic Stress Disorder.

The memories that feed Post Traumatic Stress Disorder are not always complete. They are deeply buried; so deeply, that it is difficult to recall them. This process is one the unconscious mind takes to bury bad memories. While the person with PTSD can recall the event, they often cannot remember the impact it had on their life. It is like remembering only the main course of a dinner, but not who was with you or where you at it. This unconscious process of the mind helps one avoid disquieting memories.

Now what transpires when a stimulus jars the memory deep in the unconscious? The person with PTSD will react in a manner inconsistent with the stimulus. We know for instance that our sense of smell is the most powerful of our senses. One, who has suffered trauma of fire, particularly if their home was destroyed, will react in an almost violent manner to the smell of smoke. The reactions will be just as strong whether the fire is controlled, or uncontrolled. The unconscious mind reacts to the stimulus in the same way as the conscious mind did at the time of the fire. The subconscious mind has no concept of time. As far as it is concerned, the event is happening right now. There are no modifiers in the unconscious. Every event is in the present.

If the person with PTSD has uncovered the source of the discomfort caused by certain stimuli, it is relatively simple to modify the reaction to such stimuli. As one of our associates put it, "When such an unpleasant memory comes around, simply say to yourself 'thank you for sharing that miserable situation again. Now leave.'" The idea is to recognize what causes the uneasiness and the subsequent irrational reaction. This knowledge will not make the power of mental impact, or the traumatic memory disappear. Therapy will make it understandable and tolerable. Once such unpleasantness is examined in the light of reason, it will lose a lot of its force. The process is like hearing something go bump in the night. The imagination can conjure up all sorts of frightening things. In the morning, when you find it was simply a ball that rolled down the stairs or a limb broke from a tree and hit the roof, you are relieved at the discovery. Daylight takes away the irrational reaction. Comprehension takes away the sting of previously uncovered unpleasant memories.

The problems of PTSD can be compared to the loss of a leg. If the person continued to fall down when they tried to stand up, they would soon realize they needed a crutch or an artificial limb to avoid toppling over. The debilitation caused by PTSD is not as easy to accept. The problems this disorder causes are not as obvious. Nor are the solutions as easy to recognize.

The above are simple situations that would be easy to resolve providing you had the money and capability to change them. PTSD is not so simple. The basic problem is the one who lives with PTSD often has no idea where the problem arose. In the case studies we present, you will read of the connection between the trauma, and the current day reactions to the effect of that trauma. The process of uncovering what memories the client lives with is a difficult one. It is like peeling an onion, where layer after layer of memory is uncovered until the problem at the core is discovered. The process can take a long time. A major part of the dilemma is cause by the inability of the person with PTSD to open up enough to her or him self in order to bring the long buried trauma to consciousness. Relief of the misery of PTSD can come from many directions. It could be as simple as waiting for the pain of an anniversary date, going through the seasons, or simply becoming comfortable enough with the psychotherapeutic process to allow the mental blocks to come tumbling down. There is a deep seated fear connected with the traumatic memories. Those who suffer with PTSD are unconsciously terrified of facing the situation again. Remember time is not recognized by the unconscious. So when digging around in that area of memory, there is a serious concern about looking at the reality of what occurred to cause the terrible traumatic memories.

Now, one of the strange parts of PTSD is the obtuse angle from which the unconscious memory is stimulated. For instance, men who spent a lot of time in Viet Nam, immediately remember that wartime experience upon smelling burning kerosene. That was the process used to dispose of human waste. According them, the odor was pervasive in Viet Nam. That is a pretty direct reaction, Attached to those conscious memories, can be long forgotten memories that will cause bad reactions. The smell of burning kerosene could be tied to other memories of the Viet Nam experience. Those forgotten memories, or responses, are the ones that cause the trouble. The unconscious never forgets. The reactions are triggered by memories that are apparently forgotten.

PTSD is not a phobia. If a person is afraid of reptiles, of the water, of being outside, of heights, or being confined in a small space, they can usually avoid such situations in their daily life. If the phobia is disturbing enough, or interferes with daily activities, most mental health practitioners can treat them. The difficulty with the aversions caused by PTSD is that the person does not know why they react in such a different manner than one that does not live with the results of the disorder.

ARRESTED DEVELOPMENT AND PTSD

PTSD can contribute to arrested development. We have commented on this before, and about the problems arrested development can cause. Arrested development means the actions and reactions of a teen age person in the body of an apparent developed adult. These childish actions and reactions cause confusion in the family. We hear the term "Well that's the way she (he) is about (fill in your blank), or I don't understand why she/he reacts this way. Here is a case study of one man with arrested development.

Sam is in his late 40's. He has worked most of his life for various firms as a civil engineer. Presently he is unemployed, but he expects to go back to work soon. He is in good physical health, and has no addictive habits. He and his wife of twenty five years have two children in their teens. They own their home, and are not in any financial distress.

From the outside this family appears as normal as apple pie. The husband has a good profession, his wife works part time, and the children are getting along well in their high school education process. Everyone is physically healthy.

Sam has a problem that probably began while he was an infantry soldier in Viet Nam. He celebrated his nineteenth birthday there. His military record is clean. His attitude since returning from VN has been that of a teen-age boy. He likes to play. He loves to sail on the lake near his home. He has had many affairs of short duration. He admits to no apparent planning for either his future or those of his wife and children. Because he is well regarded in his profession, he has had no problem finding work when he wants it. He is not interested in working for any one firm. He sees not problem in his extra-marital affairs, as he is in his words "very discrete." He is satisfied that he is providing shelter and food for his wife and family, so there should be no objections to his peccadilloes from them. That he is a poor role model to his children, but that does not seem to bother him at all. His attitude toward his family is one of detached interest. He has never been physically abusive.

Sam has lived with this life style and distorted perspective toward his family and occupation for so long, that we found it extremely difficult to pierce his self satisfied demeanor. We concluded that his limited outlook on his life was caused by a lack of moral development. Kohlberg's studies in this area would indicate that Sam stopped a part of his moral development in his late teens. That is the time he served in Viet Nam.

We made a number of attempts to find a single traumatic incident in his combat experience that could cause this failure to move through the egocentric attitude of a teenager to the appreciation for the lives and well being of others. Even though we cold not find a specific trauma, it is obvious his combat experience caused more than one trauma in the time in Viet Nam.

Dr. Kohlberg broke down a lifetime into three levels, child, teenager, and adult. He subdivided each level into two more stages. Sam is stuck in the first stage of being a teenager, Kohlberg's stage three, where he is aware of the norms of society, but only as they affect him. He is not willing at this stage of moral development to make efforts to help others or to assist them in their lives. He is strictly egocentric. Thus he is willing to work to support himself first, to enjoy his pleasures while apparently abiding by the standards of society, but without concern for those in his family. His concern was only about getting caught, another teen age moral standard. Because he is the authority figure by virtue of his age and family position, the fear of being caught and punished, the driving fear of the teenager, does not exist. His set of morals and ethics are strictly his.

Therapists always search for the cause of the disorder. Sometimes we cannot discover it, so we take the pragmatic attitude and simply deal with the present situation. Sam is an intelligent person with no apparent comprehension problems. So, we took the cognitive approach to resolving some of the problems between him and his family. We confronted him with his infidelities, his lack of connection with his family, his lack of reality thinking. While he did not deny these factors, he found no fault in them. Because of his attitude it took a long time for us to get through to him that his immature attitudes were causing the difficulties with his wife and children, with his failure to establish a long term occupational relationship, and his socially and morally unacceptable sexual liaison.

We in effect began a training program for a teen aged boy to become a man that would accept the social and moral standards he is expected to adhere to during his life.

DENIAL

"I don't think the war made any major differences in my life after I got out of the Army." So said Bob, a 60 year old executive, sitting in his well appointed office. He is executive vice president and chief operating officer in a mid-sized company located in the Southwest.

We met in connection with our research on the long term affects of combat and captivity on young soldiers. He was drafted as an 18 year old in World War II and served for 32 months as a sergeant in a rifle company.

During the Ardennes campaign in December 1944, two regiments of the infantry division in which he served were surrendered after being surrounded and cut off. The men of the regiments ended up in a number of prisoner of war camps scattered across Germany.

Bob and his comrades suffered humiliating defeat, physical and mental exhaustion from starvation on a diet of about 900 calories per day, and primitive medical treatment. They were liberated as the war ended, about six months after their capture. Most of the men had lost about half their body weight from the disagreeable conditions under which they survived.

After Bob was discharged from the Army, he returned home, married his childhood sweetheart, went to college and began his career. So far, so good. His life appeared normal, with only the usual upsets of living and working. In his mind, he put the POW experience behind him. He felt it had had little effect on him, other than an strong anathema toward veteran's organizations, and the Veterans Administration.

Upon questioning further, he recalled a recurring dream that had caused sleep interruption for many years. It involved a recall to his old outfit in the Army. All of the familiar faces were there, including his former company commander with whom he had disagreed violently on many occasions. He joined in a plot to kill and dispose of the captain's body. About the time he was to be caught for the crime, he would awaken in a sweat.

He admitted to drinking to excess at times, but denied he had a drinking problem. We discovered that about two years later, he had joined Alcoholic Anonymous when his drinking began to interfere with his work, and he was fired. He is now divorced. His life flew in the face of his denial.

ERNESTO

The literature on the Viet Nam war clings to the concept that the young age of the military men who served there is a major factor in their difficulty in readjustment to civilian life. There appears to be a belief that because the average age of the men fighting there was under the legal age of 21, they suffered more from the trauma of war than those who were older and in theory more mature. We do not choose to quarrel with the studies, but there are many cases we have dealt with that belie that overall conclusion.

Ernesto was a graduate of a well-regarded chiropractic college. He had practiced for two years before being drafted into the Army. The Army does not recognize any physical healers other than medical doctors. So Ernesto became a rifleman in an infantry company. He was well trained by the time he arrived in Viet Nam. He endured the same fears and trepidation of every man going in to combat. He prevailed and was decorated for his valor on the battlefield. Near the end of his tour of duty, while in a static position, he thinks he killed a woman who was trying to cross the dead line marked with concertina wire. Whether hallucinations or not, he saw her body draped over the barbed wire night and day for several days. By that time in his tour, he was extremely weary from his participation in many combat actions. He welcomed the set positions, as cover was substantial, and the artillery support was accurate. The combination of his physical fatigue and the attendant mental stress of twelve months of actions took its toll on this formerly mature and well-adjusted man. However, he did not know it for a long time.

He returned to civilian life and resumed his practice of chiropractic medicine. For many years, he had no difficulty with his memories of Viet Nam. It became as for many, a distant dream with little connection with his present life. Then the flash backs and the nightmares began.

What triggers the flash backs and the nightmares are factors we do not really understand. We have determined that they begin when the efforts to earn money and establish an agreeable position in life are better established. In this case, the sight of the inert bodies on his adjustment table began to remind him of the dead bodies after battles. He began to hallucinate about the dead woman, who he believed accompanied him wherever he went, berating him for killing her and her people. The combination of the hallucinations and the flashbacks caused by the sight of inert bodies became too much for him to continue his practice. He was still called for consultation by his professional associates. It was strange to listen to him speaking to them on the telephone, calmly and deliberately offering what appeared to us to be good medical advice. He would then come in to session, with the strange mental pictures that made face to face interpersonal treatment, and later on, simple conversation, almost impossible. He is now institutionalized for his mental condition.

NICK-ONE WE COULD NOT HELP

One of the worst cases of PTSD we know of showed up in a veteran of World War II. As we now realize, these cases then labeled "combat fatigue" would lead to PTSD in the futures of these men. Many thought that when they returned to their homes and family the past would disappear to be replaced with the normalcy of civilian life. Peaceful surroundings with family and friends were supposed to eliminate the horrors of war experiences. The doctors in World War I had disproved this (see the Rivers commentary elsewhere in this book.)

Our subject who we will call Nick was in his late 60's when we first met him. He had worked all of his life in the construction trades, and had retired to enjoy his golden years in a retirement community in Arizona. He had never been a social person, so his number of friends was very limited. He could not read, a fact he had managed to overcome in a trade that demanded the ability to read blueprints and specifications. Now, he could no longer work, even part time, because of the physical deterioration caused by age.

Because he could not read, his major past time was watching television. War movies disturbed him. In an effort to eliminate this problem, he forced himself to watch some of them. The effort was disastrous. Nightmares of the war returned with such force that his wife had to move into another bedroom. Flashbacks happened with such regularity that he thought he was losing his mind. He began to withdraw, became paranoid even with members of his family, and no longer involved himself in community activities. He became increasingly disturbed by his illiteracy. Because he could not read, he had no knowledge of the help available to him as an Army veteran. His personal physician who had found no organic problems when he examined Nick referred him to us for therapy.

The hardships of war seemed to be accepted by men such as Nick who were raised in the Great Depression. War was just another time of privation, physical effort, and the adversity they had learned to accept and deal with during their youth. When the post World War II years brought steady work, and personal prosperity, that combination caused the trauma of wartime to disappear in the routine of every day life. None of these war veterans realized the time bomb ticking in their unconscious that would cause them grief in their later years.

He saw his terrible discomfort as simply another difficult time in his life. We could never get through the shell he had built around himself which was created by the self-loathing brought on in the main from survival guilt. He had managed to live through some horrible battles. In one that lasted many days, he used the bodies of his comrades to protect himself from enemy fire. That nightmare came back often.

Other nightmares are of terrible fear, being surrounded, and trying to run. He is withdrawn from society. This withdrawal became a problem when he retired. He became more and more withdrawn. His interest in living diminished. He was frustrated and angry. His specific memory of events is poor as the result of selective amnesia. He spoke of his wounds as though they happened to someone else.

We lost track of Nick when he never returned for more therapy. Mail to him was returned. These are the tragedies of PTSD. A man who did his job both as a husband and father, and accepted his duty to country, continues to live with the nightmares of battle that echo in his mind day and night. While he deserves to live in comfort and peace for the rest of his days, he cannot because of the damage done to his psyche during his childhood and in time of war.

AFRICAN AMERICAN SOLDIERS IN SOMALIA

An unexpected source of PTSD was the military work in Somalia, particularly for the black men in uniform. In spite of the efforts of the military to eliminate bigotry and separation, the soldier of color continues to feel different. Many of them went to Somalia with the feeling they would help bring order and peace to a troubled area, primarily a Black Country. Instead, they found bigotry and hatred from the Somalis who could not and did not allow our men to feel as though they were helping people with a common culture. The people of Somalia thought of them as the hated Americans, who had no concern for the fate of the native Somalis. This final rejection caused great problems with nightmares and flashbacks among these men who have lived with feelings of rejection for generations.

SEAN

Sean J., a 19 year old Army sergeant, was a helicopter waist gunner on in Viet Nam. On a mission during the invasion of Cambodia, the group ran into heavy ground fire. The pilots in Sean's helicopter were killed, as was the other gunner. Realizing the bird was going to crash, Sean bailed out when he was still about 200 feet in the air. He was still awake when he hit the ground. Realizing that he was close to the enemy positions, he crawled further into the jungle to hide. He lost consciousness from the pain of multiple injuries to his spine and internal organs. When the rescue squad came in to recover the bodies, they realized there was one man, or body, missing. They wee able to find Sean and evacuate him to a field hospital. He was later moved to a hospital in Japan, and then to Letterman Hospital at the Presidio in California.

Recovery from his wounds and subsequent therapy took two years. He was medically discharged from the Army. The medics told him he would probably be able to walk for about five years, and then he would be confined to a wheel chair for the rest of his life. During this time, he attempted suicide. He was 22 years old.

Sean was able to work at a number of jobs in civilian life, but in about five years, his physical condition forced him to quit working. In the past fifteen years or so, he has undergone three more major surgeries on his spinal cord. He is able to move around well, but tires easily. He is married, but has no children.

Sean lives with all of the symptoms of Post Traumatic Stress Disorder. While he is socially active, he prefers to be alone. Paranoia is constant. He often awakens in the night feeling that his house is being watched, or someone is attempting entry.

Sean sleeps fitfully. In many years he has not had a complete night's rest. He may stay awake for 36 hours, and then nap intermittently for three or four days. His interrupted sleep pattern is in part the result of nightmares, and the subsequent concern they will return. Part of his sleeplessness is due to pain from his wounds and surgeries, but much of it is from the trauma of lying in a jungle, wounded, helpless and alone. The inability to relax is a direct result of the need to be alert to danger resulting from the trauma of the crash.

While Sean is a socially active, his friends are limited to those who served in Viet Nam, and one or two childhood friends. He maintains a personal reserve that is not penetrable. Again, the result of surviving alone. The reactions to a combat situation continue in civilian life years later.

While Sean avoids experiences that would remind him of Viet Nam, he does work as a volunteer in a Veterans Administration clinic. He gets personal satisfaction from helping others who need assistance in living with their own set of demons. The effects of his personal experiences in combat, and recovering from his wounds in a VA hospital, are invaluable in helping others who continue to feel helpless and hopeless. He has volunteered at this task for a number of years, but in the past two years or so his interest in this activity is lessening.

Sean also has a desire to live simply, and in restricted areas. While his home is spacious, he would feel better if he were in a smaller home or condominium. This too results from the fears deeply seated in his subconscious as the result of the helicopter crash, and the lengthy periods of hospitalization during which he was helpless and exposed. These feelings are not an indication of lack of courage, but fears that seem groundless except to the experienced psychotherapist.

Sean lives with some flashbacks which take him back to Viet Nam in an instant. One that recurs more often than others is the memory of falling past the green of the jungle trees. The duration of that experience could not have been more than a few seconds as he bailed out of the helicopter from less than 300 feet. Other unpleasant memories revolve around missions in the helicopter squadron, or from rocket attacks while on the ground. These intrusive memories are less frequent now than ten or fifteen years ago, but are as intense as ever. Therapy has helped Sean live with the results of these offensive replays of traumatic incidents, but they continue to leave him shaken for the moment.

For years on the anniversary of the crash, he was unable to leave his house. With therapy, he found the courage at first to use the telephone, and then walk out into the yard, and now can face the day without the former uncontrollable panic that immobilized him. The anniversary day is not without misgivings and disquietude, but he knows where the feelings come from and can live with them now.

So we see in this situation, a young man, seriously wounded, and still suffering from the physical after effects of his wounds. He also lives with the effects of Post Traumatic Stress Disorder as the result of the trauma of war, and the intensity of the final battle in which he was involved. The battle continues with his fears (definitely not cowardice), his feelings of a foreshortened future, his increasing unwillingness to become involved with others, some difficulty in completing tasks, and continuing anxiety. The consequences of his physical and mental wounding are synergistic. He lives with a mental uncertainty of a foreshortened physical future because of his wounding, which is exacerbated by the same feelings from his PTSD. Sean truly has more than double trouble in his life because of the combination of these two problems.

FORMER PRISONERS OF WAR

There are many difficulties with former prisoners of war. Many of them are loners, with a distant manner. They find social intercourse difficult. Many took jobs that kept them out of crowds, allowing them to function well without the pressures of others. Many former prisoners of war live with a well disguised anger, which comes to the fore when values held closely are questioned or discounted. They live with the frugality learned from lack of food and other basic life needs. Many suffer nightmares when reminded of their combat or prisoner of war experiences. They live with the hyper alertness, and sometimes feelings of helplessness and hopelessness caused by incarceration as a prisoner of war.

Because they were exposed to events outside the range of human experience, armed military combat, and incarceration as a prisoner of war, both extreme stressors have led to Post Traumatic Stress Disorder and all of its ramifications including limiting the joy of living.

Francois Ambriere who was a prisoner of war for almost five years wrote in The Long Holiday: (1948) these words where he unknowingly described the source of PTSD for the former captive.

> Something of it will live on in the memories and hearts of those who experienced it (captivity). The camp never does vanish. The memories are potent and deep seated in the compartment of the mind reserved for the time spent there. After years one no longer remembers why, but wonders about actions taken and

situations avoided that relate to old privation and suffering. (p. vii). [15]

Dr. Robert Obourn, who was a Veterans Administration psychiatrist, himself a former prisoner of war described the situation:

> A Prisoner of War is a mission failed. The ex-Prisoner of War lives with a sense of embarrassment. The tradition of the American Armed Services is one of pride and success. The POW cannot share in this. Although not his fault, having been a POW is a source of quiet embarrassment. POW's are quiet men and women, who seem very tolerant of the world around them. [16]

What he did not say, because PTSD had not yet been determined to be the aftermath of combat and captivity, is that the "sense of embarrassment" would turn into Post Traumatic Stress Disorder in the later years of their lives. Dr. Viktor Frankl who spent almost four years in a concentration camp summed up the problem best in these few words: "No explanations are needed for those who have been inside, and the others will understand neither how we felt then nor how we feel now." (1984, p. 24). [5]

POLITICAL REFUGEES

Political refugees live with PTSD. They have survived the destruction of their way of life. They have lived through not only the loss of the home and society in which they lived, but also the revolution and destruction that surrounded that loss. People who were in positions of power and authority found themselves on the run and at the mercy of the new power structure. They have told us about their continuing and unreasonable fear of authority that developed from the trauma of dealing with bureaucrats who controlled their lives after the revolution ended. The freedom in their lives disappeared with all of the other trappings of comfort of their former life style. They now have a fear of closed spaces--not claustrophobia, but rather a great discomfort in not being able to get free of any kind of restrictions. An uneasy dichotomy exists between the concern for safety, which requires locked quarters, and the dread of restricted spaces. Loud noises, especially helicopters flying over head and the explosions on the Fourth of July create uneasiness beyond the cognitive acceptance of the harmlessness of the racket. One Middle Eastern refugee told us of the terror created in her mind when she heard the sounds of mock battle at a nearby military base. Rational thought does little good when the unconscious mind has returned to the days of revolution and strife swirling around one's home.

Some of these fears are passed on to the children. One survivor told us her unreasonable concern for the safety of her children when they were not with her probably came from her father's fears for the family during revolutionary times. He was greatly disturbed when the children were out of the house for any reason, no matter how innocent or apparently safe their destination.

THE SCANDAVIAN PSYCHIATRIST

A psychiatrist who lived through the occupation of Norway during World War II asked us once why we thought he had PTSD. The family was able to remain in their home, and as far as he could remember, his parents had no problems with the occupying army. He said he had no memory of difficulty during that time. He was a schoolboy in his early teens during that time. His father was a railroad supervisor who went to work every day as he always had. There were no discussions between his parents about the occupation. It was in his words "As though everything was as it always had been." Yet, he lived with the classic symptoms of hyperalertness, nighmares, flashbacks, and a feeling of being different some way.

When we met him, he was involved in University studies of captivity and torture in modern times and was a recognized authority in that field. In the main, the studies investigated wartime incidents in Nazi Germany and the occupied countries. They also researched present day events particularly in the Pol Pot regime in Cambodia, the atrocities in Bosnia, and the continuing dehumanization in the gulags.

We asked him to look into his unconscious to determine the reasons for his deep and abiding interest in the anguish of the captive. It was our opinion that the tension felt by his parents was transmitted to him in many subtle ways, often enough so that on some deep level he too lived with the unspoken terrors they felt. In addition, his interest in captivity and torture did not spring full grown in his university days. We suggested that it was an outgrowth of his youth, during which he was aware of his whole country living in captivity and that innocent people suffered torment and the tribulations of being subservient to an outside power. In this case, we see PTSD without any personal violent trauma, but rather the cumulative effect of a national trauma as from the brutality of war time occupation forces.

EFFECTS OF POST TRAUMATIC STRESS ON SECOND GENERATIONS

We have observed PTSD in the second generation of those who lived with the terrible trauma of the Holocaust. We are acquainted with two intelligent, outwardly well adjusted young women. Both of their parents are survivors of Auschwitz. They exhibited some of the aspects of Post Traumatic Stress Disorder. One was their inability to make close associations with others, even with each other, and certainly with their parents. They were constantly alert to any imagined slight, and lived with well developed paranoia. Both of them had apparently normal eating habits. On one occasion, we invited them for dinner. While serving the soup course to them, one requested that we just "Skim some off of the top." In the concentration camps, in order to get more nourishment, prisoners asked the server to "Scoop from the bottom of the soup pot." The other woman would only take half portions. These young women's requests could have been dictated by a desire for a slim body. We felt it was a conditioned response learned as a child at their dinner table. The parents needed (and continued to exhibit the now unneeded) better nutrition in order to survive in the camps.

Post Traumatic Stress Disorder is almost a given condition in those who were held in concentration camps, gulags, and in POW camps. As the field of psychology worked with these people, more and more understanding of the condition itself, and methods of treatment to alleviate it evolved. Forgotten in the process were the sons and daughters and spouses of those who had undergone such incarceration. One concentration camp survivor said "We can only apologize to our children and hope they will some day understand the devils that should have been long ago buried, but continue to disturb our lives."

In the MGM picture "Homecoming" made in the late 1940's, Clark Gable played An Army surgeon returning from three years of wartime service. He was asked by a correspondent if he had a story to tell of his experience. Gable's character demurs, saying, "No one at home would want to hear it anyway." The correspondent replies "You are wrong. They are the ones who will have to live with us when we get home. They need to know what happened to us in war." He did not say, nor probably did not understand how much talking about the experiences might help one who had lived through wartime horror.

Those who did not live through the same experience will never understand those who lived under the cruelty of the camps. The responsibility to avoid passing on the neuroses developed for survival falls squarely on those who went through such trauma. The lessons learned are of little value in civilian peacetime life. The mental gyrations necessary for survival under these horrible circumstances are often forced upon the children, or spouses, who learn to react to situations in the same distorted manner as the one with PTSD.

There is a time for silence in our daily lives. There was a more serious need for silence in armed combat. One avoided excess noise to keep positions hidden from the enemy. In the camps, one kept silent to avoid the guard's attention. Those who were in the camps learned to remain still and silent, lest they be picked for extra work details. Sometimes they were picked out for a beating for no reason other than the guards looked for a victim. Those who moved or made a noise were obvious targets. Families of those who lived with that fear are forced to live with a greater silence than others. Children do not understand why their parent insists they maintain a generally quiet decorum when their friends do not live with such restrictions. We found that once we pointed out to our client what he or she was doing to their family, especially the children, they were willing to forgo this former excessive need for quiet in the house. Most all had forgotten why they made the demand. Many of them did tell us that while they accepted the recommendation, they remained uncomfortable with any kind of noise level.

These cases of Post Traumatic Stress are not the result of the traditional definitions as outlined in the DSMIV. None of these cases involved "direct personal experience of an event that involves actual or threatened death or serious injury, or other threat to one's physical integrity; or witnessing an event that involves death, injury, or a threat to the physical integrity of another person." (DSMIV). Rather they are the result of early teachings by parents who lived with full blown PTSD from their terrifying experiences and trauma. The children are totally unaware they are reacting to traumas suffered in some cases before they were born.

We can only wonder how many generations will live with the behavioral restrictions learned so painfully by survivors of the concentration camps of Nazi Germany.

SURVIVOR OF A ROCKET ATTACK

A career Navy man was stationed on the Stark, a US Navy destroyer attacked by the Iraqi Air Force during the Gulf War. He had been the unofficial alcohol counselor on the ship as he had many years in recovery from alcoholism. He had helped many men with their sobriety program during that time.

The Iraqi aircraft fired Silk rockets, which tore a huge hole in the ship, killing seventeen men in one compartment. Because our client had had a lot of experience in counseling, he was asked to help in the survivors in that compartment. He was among the first men to enter the badly destroyed area of the ship. According to his description, the carnage was unbelievable. Some the bodies were totally unidentifiable as the result of the explosion and subsequent fire, all of the bodies were badly mangled, and some were just parts. Not only did our man suffer the trauma of spending a lot of time in the area that had been damaged on the ship but he lived with the fear that either the ship would sink because of the damage to it, or suffer another attack. He was torn between his duty and desire to help the survivors, and the impact of the horrible scene.

The fear he experienced when he moved into area of death and destruction continued to as he worked with survivors of the attack and other members of the crew. This man was asked to do more than he had been trained for. His ability to work with addictive people had not prepared him to deal with the intense emotions caused by this unexpected and violent attack on the ship. Research in these area shows that the non-volunteers in cases of body recovery have a greater predisposition to PTSD than does the professional undertaker. Our man was among the non-volunteers. His subsequent PTSD was a direct result of this trauma.

MILITARY NON COMBATANTS INCUR PTSD

We are inclined to think that PTSD only results from being physically involved in, or observing a traumatic incident. The psychological community, as indicated in the descriptions in the DSMIV, has recognized the effect that witnessing the death or serious injury of another can create PTSD. Only once did we see a serious case of Post Traumatic Stress Disorder where neither of the foregoing conditions existed. This involved a record clerk whose job it was to review the personnel files of fatal casualties during the Viet Nam war. This man was stationed in Japan. He never got near the war zone. He came to us describing sleep disturbances, isolation, and nightmares, all indicating PTSD. We were puzzled by our own diagnosis, as we could not find any trauma in his background that could have created the disorder. There was no indication of any premorbidity. After a lot of discussion, we realized the man had in fact suffered trauma from the months of review of the event and conditions surrounding their deaths. He began to internalize the circumstances surrounding the deaths. Without realizing it, his imagination began to work on his unconscious. The deaths of these men became real to him. They were not pages in a file. His memory retained the hundreds of death events. Consciously, he felt he was leaving the details of his work when he left the office. But his unconscious could not let go.

Upon his return to civilian life, he did not ruminate on his work while overseas. But almost like clockwork, when he got into his forties, the unconscious memories came back, and created the same effect on his life as if he had been in combat. In his case, it was worse, as every day he was dealing with the deaths of young men. The horror of war was transferred to his mind by the review of file after file that contained the details of the violent death of men and women. His problem was exacerbated by his belief that he should have not had any continuing problems from his duty as he never was in a combat zone. He felt that because he had not seen combat, he had little in common with those who had and now lived with the aftereffects of that experience.

Many have difficulty in understanding the power of the unconscious. This man's unconscious mind had a long column of the dead marching through it. The letters to the surviving family contained in the files increased his pain. The survivor guilt he felt was intensified because he had never been exposed to danger. We were able to show him the latent power of the work he had done in the military and to minimize his feelings that he was in some way inadequate.

In other non-combat situations that caused PTSD researchers found that a professional mortuary worker was better able to handle single body casualties of war in the Gulf, than those who were inexperienced. The most affected was the non-volunteer mortuary worker. Symptoms of PTSD were more pronounced in those who handled the highest numbers of remains. Those who handled the bodies after an explosion on a Navy ship reported more intrusion, avoidance, and hostility than did non-body handlers. We know from the research, that exposure to traumatic death increases the risk of PTSD.

NATURAL DISASTERS-VOLCANO ERUPTION

Vern worked in the Philippines as an engineer for a major international company. His major responsibility was supervising the communications personnel, and maintaining the communications equipment. A volcano erupted, dumping about three feet of volcanic ash on the base from which the firm was operating. All but a few of the more than 600 people on the base, including Vern's family, were removed to Australia. Vern and his staff were needed to maintain contact with the home base there. What had been an active, well-populated area became almost a ghost town. Vacations from the job were eliminated because there was only a skeleton crew. The isolation and discomfort were overwhelming. Everyone was still recovering from the trauma created when the volcano erupted. Shortages of spare parts created almost constant crises. The niceties of life to which these overseas employees had become accustomed were limited. Their families were gone. The theater and the gourmet restaurant were both closed. No hazard pay was authorized. The volcano continued to smoke, polluting the air, causing respiratory and vision problems. The men remaining felt like prisoners who had lived through a terrible trauma now exacerbated by their present physical distress and discomfort.

After the company brought Vern out of the area, he began to have nightmares about being buried under the volcanic ash. Part of that we thought was the retained memory of the volcanic gas odor. We know that the sense of smell continues long after any other senses have been dulled. He has another continuing nightmare where he continues to dig in the volcanic ash trying to get to his family who are buried in it. He felt totally helpless as he searched for them in the featureless gray expanse. His nightmares also involved thinking his family was buried in the volcanic ash, but because of the rain which turned it almost into concrete, he could not get to them.

As a result of the loneliness and feelings of separation from the world, Vern developed paranoia. He saw danger all over. The loss of the stability of his company, the feeling of abandonment when the forced him and a few others to remain in a desolate and uninhabited area contributed to his unconscious feelings that someone was out to get him. He clung to the stability inherent in his wife. He became almost unemployable but because of his reputation, and skills he was able to work only on a part time basis. He held many jobs, a situation attributable to his inability to get along with his fellow workers. He was never fired. Often he had supervisory jobs, but the responsibility soon became too much for him to handle, in part because of his sleepless nights, and he would leave.

LONELINESS AND WITHDRAWAL

One client who had been a prisoner of war described his feelings while in the camps. "We suffered from loneliness --an indescribably deep loneliness. Our loneliness was an essence, the distillation of being alone and abandoned. We became children lost from parents. Separated forever from dead comrades and from those who disappeared during captivity. During withdrawal to save ourselves, we built a protection in loneliness that remained with us. Our loneliness became a way of life. We learned to love it as a friend."

Part of his PTSD expressed itself in his feelings of aloneness. The diagnosis of the disorder sets out the feelings of being different, and not having good interpersonal relations. We could see the effect of his captivity in his preset life. He equated loneliness with survival. Survival is most important to us all. He lived with that feeling for so long that it became part of his psyche, making it almost impossible to become close to another person.

Combining the problems caused by PTSD such as arrested development narcissism, and self-centeredness, it seems that an effort to get outside of oneself is an important factor in learning to live with the effects of Post Traumatic Stress Disorder.

William C. Menninger, MD of the famed Menninger Clinic sets out his criteria to measure emotional maturity:

- An ability to deal constructively with reality.

- The capacity to adapt to change.

- A relative freedom from symptoms that are produced by tensions and anxieties.

- The capacity to find more satisfaction in giving than receiving.

- The capacity to relate to other people in a consistent manner with mutual satisfaction and helpfulness

- The capacity to sublimate, to direct one's instinctive hostile energy into creative and constructive outlets.

- The capacity to love.

Interestingly, many others including Dr. Viktor Frankl, Dr. Carl Jung, and Bill Wilson have set out these factors for inner peace. All of them involve a concern for others more than self.

MULTIPLE PERSONALITY DISORDER AND PTSD

Working with those who live with the difficulties of PTSD raises questions for researchers to investigate further. One of those is Multiple Personality Disorder. Any number of individual personalities living in one person evidences that disorder.

From the empirical evidence we have seen in many cases of PTSD, we think there is a definite connection between it and Multiple Personality Disorder. The effects of trauma seem to fix a time in the person's life. This is most obvious in war veterans who connect their sexual experiences in a war zone with their peacetime lives years later. Among the most obvious and sensitive area is in sexual experiences, which may have started with prostitutes. Those feelings involved only immediate gratification. This early exposure and experience sticks with the person when he becomes involved someone who he loves an entirely different manner. Unfortunately, the experience leaves a deep impression that will not allow the husband to approach his wife in the tender and loving manner he would choose. This can lead to many difficult situations outside of the wedding bed and beyond the immediate sexual relationships of a man and wife.

DRUG THERAPY

We feel it important to mention the drugs used to offset mental disturbance. As psychotherapists we cannot prescribe drugs for our clients. That function is reserved for the medical profession. There are many modern drugs that have proved effective in alleviating PTSD and other mental problems. However, it is our opinion that too often the medications merely mask the problems. The positive factor is the use of such drugs in minimizing symptoms that may prove too disturbing for the client to address.

Drugs have the same affect as when physical pain interferes with treatment. The use of modern pain-killers has speeded healing after surgery. Others may help in comfortable living with chronic pain when there is no process for eliminating the problem.

THE BRIGHT SPOTS IN PTSD

Dasberg (1987) writes:

> The stress of the Holocaust has taught us that human beings can undergo extreme traumatic experiences, become deeply impaired and yet still retain the ability to rehabilitate their ego forces. They continue to have an increased vulnerability to stress

situations, but also a greater sensitivity towards fellow humans a greater capacity for empathy and a greater appreciation for the higher values in life. 3

We think this heightened sensitivity is the result of learning about oneself, by uncovering the hidden drives that run our lives. In so doing one can recognize there is pain that others live with, even though they did not experience the types of trauma that causes Post Traumatic Stress Disorder.

A FINAL WORD ABOUT PTSD-YOURS OR SOMEONE ELSES

Do not look for Post Traumatic Stress Disorder in your life unless you are confused as to why you are disturbed by living, your family, fellow workers, and all of society. Look inside yourself if you are experiencing nightmares; having uncomfortable and inopportune flashbacks to a trauma in your past. Check to see if you are living with disturbing memories that crowd into your consciousness at the most inappropriate times; and feeling that life has no meaning any longer so that you may as well not live each day to its fullest. Then take yourself to a professional who can sort out superficial feelings of frustration and the normal problems of living from the agony of PTSD. There is help to alleviate these distorted reactions to life events now. We wish you and your loved ones well in your search for inner peace.

APPENDIX 1

The following is an abridgment of the description of Post Traumatic Stress Disorder as outlined in the Diagnostic and Statistical Manual of the American Psychiatric Association, version 3.0 Copyright American Psychiatric Publishing Group (Washington DC) 1994-1998.

The essential feature of Post Traumatic Stress Disorder is the development of characteristic symptoms following exposure to an extreme traumatic stressor involving personal experience of an event that involves actual or threatened death or serious injury, or other threat to one's physical integrity. Or the witnessing of an event that involves death, injury, or a threat to the physical integrity of another person. The symptoms can result from learning about unexpected or violent death, serious harm, or threat of death or injury experienced by a family member or other close associate. The person's response to the event involves intense fear, helplessness, or horror.

Symptoms resulting from such traumatic events include persistent re-experiencing of the traumatic event; persistent avoidance of reminders associated with the trauma which can create persistent symptoms of increased arousal; and the strange dichotomy with those symptoms, a numbing of general responsiveness. These symptoms cause distress or impairment in social, occupational, or other important areas of functioning.

Traumatic events that are experienced directly include, military combat, violent personal assault (sexual assault, physical attack, robbery, mugging), terrorist attack, torture, incarceration as a prisoner of war or in a concentration camp, natural or manmade disasters, severe automobile accidents, or being diagnosed with a life-threatening illness. sexual experiences without threatened or actual violence or injury.

Witnessed events include, observing the serious injury or unnatural death of another person due to violent assault, accident, war, or disaster or unexpectedly witnessing a dead body or body parts.

Events experienced by others that are learned about include, but are not limited to, violent personal assault, serious accident, or serious injury experienced by a family member or a close friend; learning about the sudden, unexpected death of a family member or a close friend; or learning that one's child has a life-threatening disease.

The traumatic event can be re-experienced in various ways. Commonly the person has recurrent and intrusive recollections of the event or recurrent distressing dreams during which the event is replayed. Sometimes the person experiences dissociative states that last from a few seconds to several hours, during which components of the event are relived and the person behaves as though experiencing the event at that moment (flashbacks). Psychological distress or physiological reactivity can occur when the person is exposed to triggering events that resemble or symbolize an aspect of the traumatic event (intrusive memories.)

The person commonly makes efforts to avoid thoughts, feelings, or conversations about the traumatic event and to avoid activities, situations, or people who arouse recollections of it. This avoidance may include amnesia for an important aspect of the traumatic event. "Psychic numbing" or "emotional anesthesia" usually begins soon after the traumatic event. The individual may complain of having markedly diminished interest or participation in previously enjoyed activities, of feeling detached or estranged from other people, or of having markedly reduced ability to feel emotions (especially those associated with intimacy, tenderness, and sexuality). The individual may have a sense of a foreshortened future.

The individual has persistent symptoms of anxiety or increased arousal that were not present before the trauma. These symptoms may include difficulty falling or staying asleep that may be due to recurrent nightmares during which the traumatic event is relived, hype vigilance, and exaggerated startle response. Some individuals report irritability or outbursts of anger or difficulty concentrating or completing tasks.

REFERENCES

1. Bussbaum, Yitzak (1994) *Life and Teachings of Hillel*, New York, Jason Aaronson
2. Father Phillip Blake S.J. (1996) Lectures at Retreat House, Los Altos CA.
3. Dasberg, Lea as quoted by Campel, Yolanda Jounal of the American Academy of Psychotherapy, Guilford Putlications Fall 1998.
4. Semprum, Jorge (1980). *What a beautiful Sunday.* California: Harcourt, Brace and Jovanovich.
5. Maurel, Micheline (1958). *An ordinary camp.* New York: Simon and Schuster.
6. Frankl, Viktor, MD (1946). *Man's search for meaning.* New York: Simon & Shuster.
7. Williams, Eric Ernest (1949). *The wooden horse.* New York: Harper & Bros.
8. Pyle, Ernie (1944) *Brave men.* New York: Henry Holt.
9. Miller, Judith (1990). *One by one by one.* New York: Simon & Schuster.
10. Des Pres, Terrence (1976). *The survivor.* New York: Oxford Press.
11. Whiting, Charles (1984). *Ardennes.* London: Century Publishing.
12. Wentzel, Fritz (1954). *Single or return?* London: William Kimber.
13. Jones and Cherry(1988) Grief Recovery Handbook. New York: Harper & Rowe..
14. Manchester, William (1979) *American Caesar.* New York: Dell Publishing.
15. Ambiere, Francis (1948). *The long holiday.* Chicago: Ziff-Davis.

16. Obourn, Robert L., MD (1988, August) *Post Traumatic stress disorder and the POW.* Presented at Ex-POW MedSearch Seminar DAV Building, Kansas City, MO. In Ex-POW Bulletin.
17. DSMIV Practice Guidelines of the American Psychiatric Association. (1997): Washington DC.

SUBJECT INDEX

Affects of PTSD, 63
Ambiere, Francois, 143
An Out of Phase Disorder, 17
Anger, 65
Anniversary Date Problems, 85
Arrested Development and PTSD, 48, 72,130
Avoidance, 39, 55
Blake SJ, Fr. Philip, 18, 115
Cases, iii, 127
Causes of Upset, 59
Causes of PTSD, 1, 75
Characteristics, 29
Communication Techniques, 98
Coping, 97
Denial, 133
Distorted Memory, 37
Distorted Perception of PTSD, 15
Do I Have PTSD? 13
Dreams and Nightmares 52
Drug Therapy,157
Effect of PTSD on the Second Generation, 147
Emotional Stability Inventory, 107
Feelings of Loss, 113
Flashbacks, 33, 89
Frankl, Dr. Viktor, 22, 44, 163
Freud, Dr. Sigmund, v
German Army Hospital Ship, 88
Guilt and Inadequacy, 93
Hyper-alertness, 39
Intrusive Memories, iv, 68
Lack of Caring, 24, 38
Learned Helplessness, 56
Loneliness and Withdrawal, 91, 154

Look at Yourself, 105
Loss of Innocence, 30
MacArthur, Gen. 116
Maslow A. 67
Misdiagnosis of PTSD, 22
Multiple Personality Disorder and PTSD, 156
Narcissism and Egocentricity, 44
Natural Disasters, 153
Non-Combatants and PTSD, 151
Norwegian Ferry, 88
Out of Phase Disorder 17
Principles to Live By, 110
Political Refugees, 144
Prisoners of War, 143
Psychic Numbing, 70, 160
Railroad Disease, i
Repression, i, ii
Rivers, W. H., Capt., i
Sex, 68
Shipwrecks, 85
Somalia, 139
Strange Behavior Patterns, 47
Suspicion, 44
Test for PTSD, 13, 63
The Scandinavian Psychiatrist, 146
The Value of Therapy, 119
To Therapists, 121
Trauma defined, 4
Unwillingness to Talk About Trauma, 35
War Veterans, 94
What Else You Can Do For Yourself, 123
What to Look For, 23

Other material available from Consultors, Inc..

THE LIBERATION OF STALAG IXB, Germany.
Motion pictures taken at Stalag IXB in April 1945. Actual black and white film of the camp after liberation. . . live.
Ten Minute Silent Video tape. $19.95. plus $2. S&H.

PHOTOGRAPHS. American Prisoners of War, and Prison Camps. An album of black and white photos taken at Stalags IXA, IXB, IVB, and XIIA before, during and after WWII. *Photo book.* $18.95. plus $2. S&H

HEALING THE CHILD WARRIOR, A Search for Inner Peace. By Richard Peterson. The story of a journey back to the battlefields and German prison camps to find understanding of the long-term effects of combat and captivity on young soldiers from many countries during WWII,. Korea, and Viet Nam..

Order from: Consultors, Inc, 1285 Rubenstein Avenue Cardiff by the Sea, CA 92007   760-632-1213
Visa and M/C accepted.
Print date 5-05-03